Essentials in Hip and Ankle

Edited by Carlos Suarez-Ahedo, Anell Olivos-Meza and Arie M. Rijke

Published in London, United Kingdom

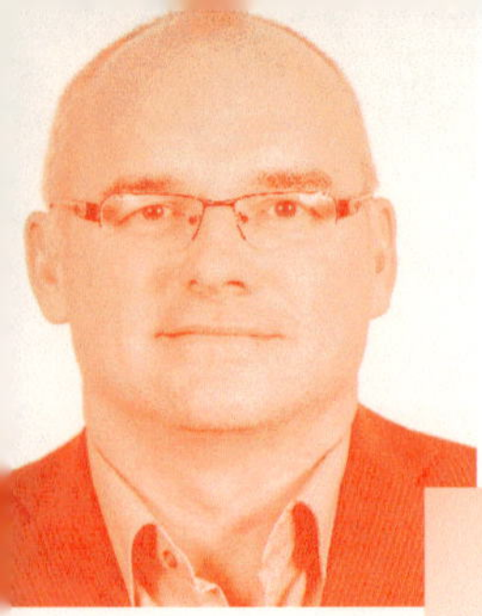
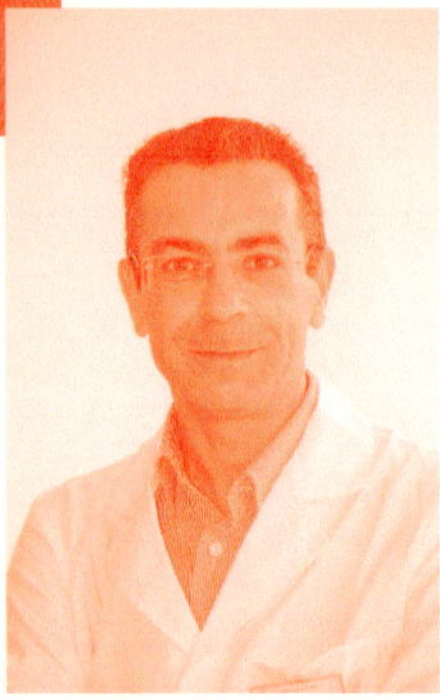
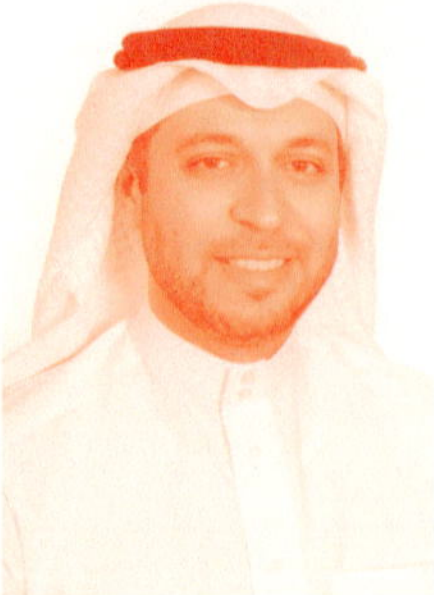
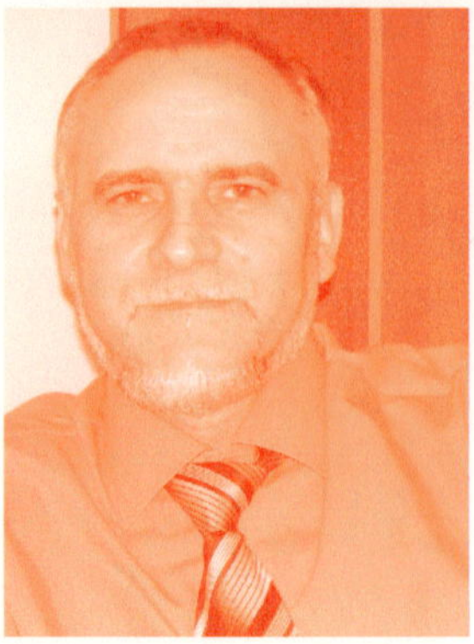
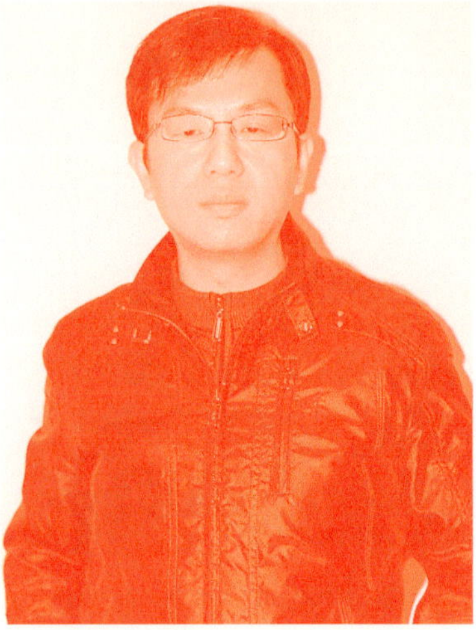
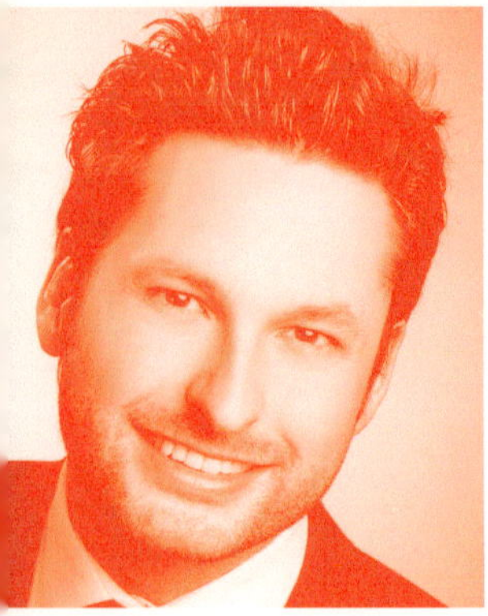
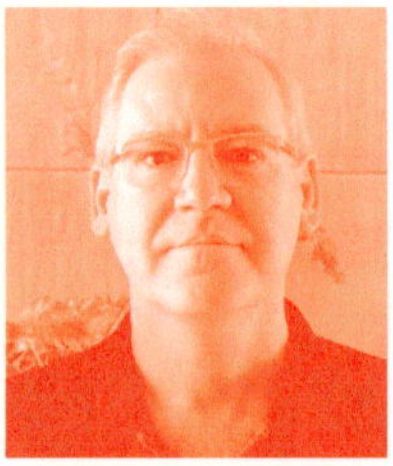

IntechOpen

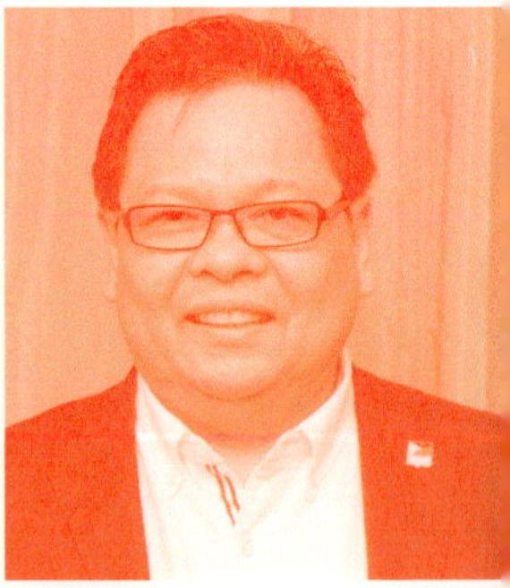
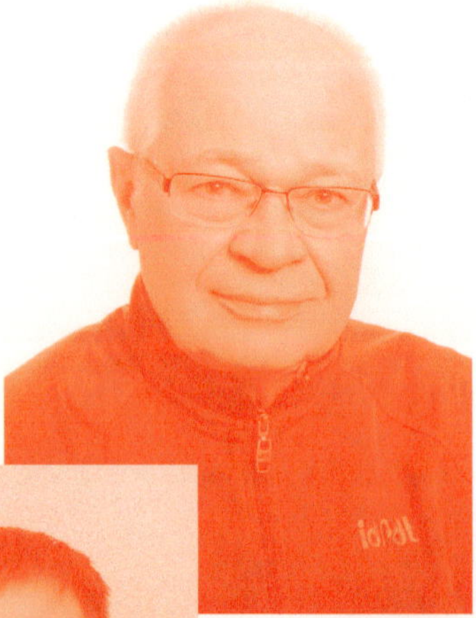
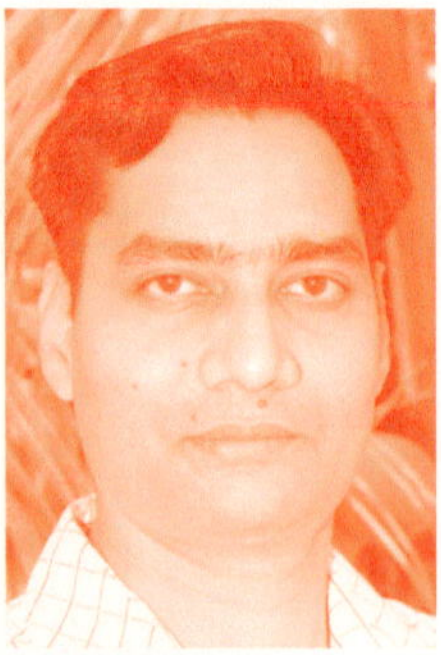
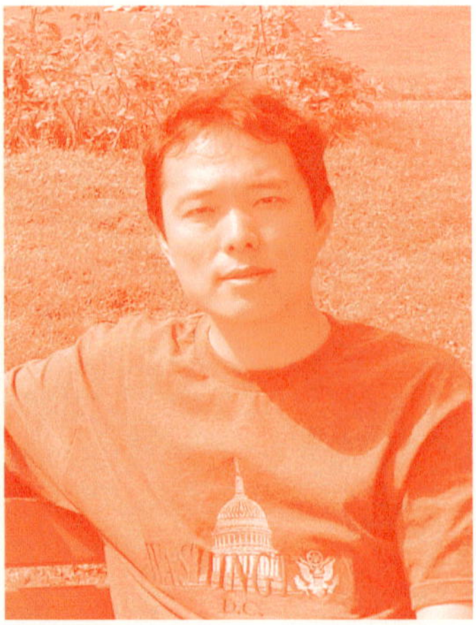
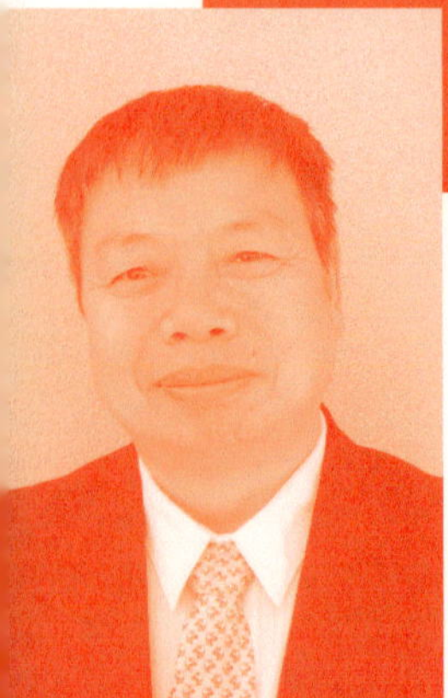
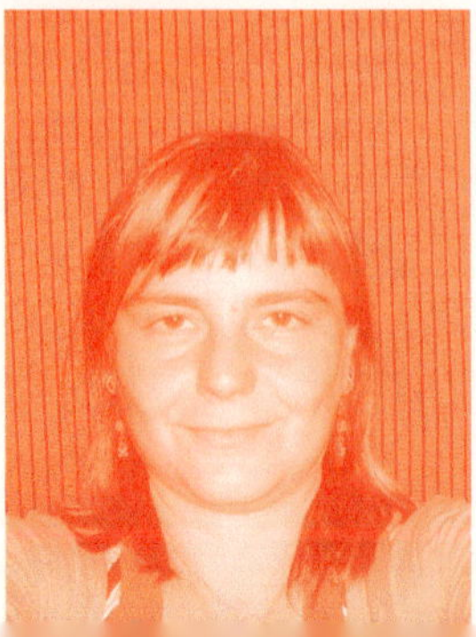

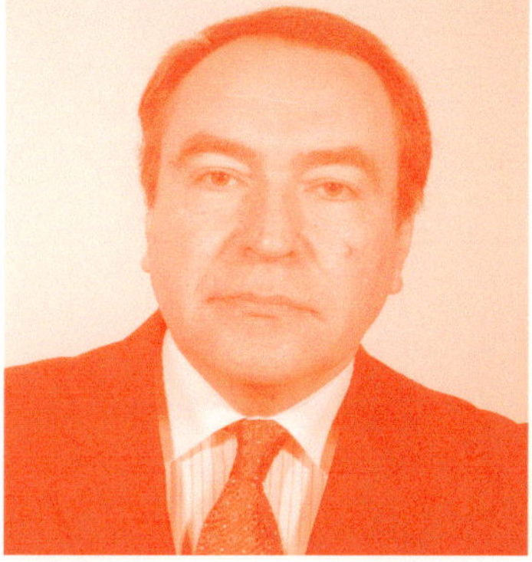
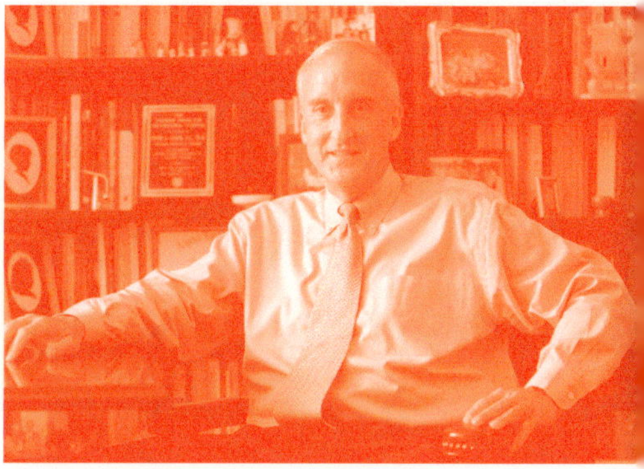
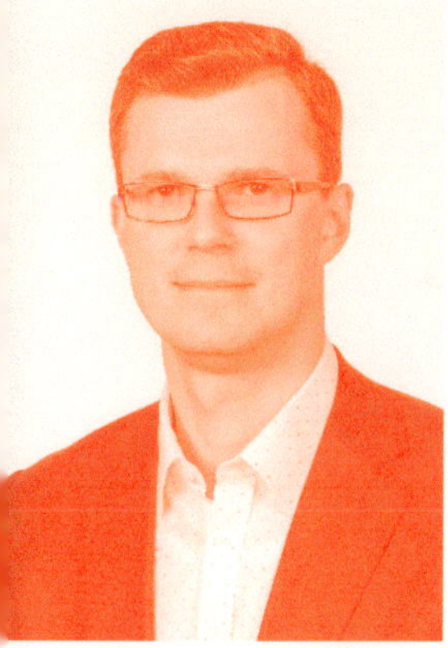
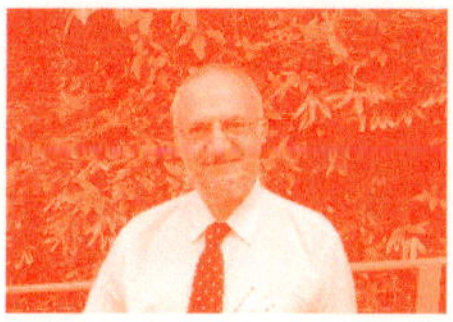
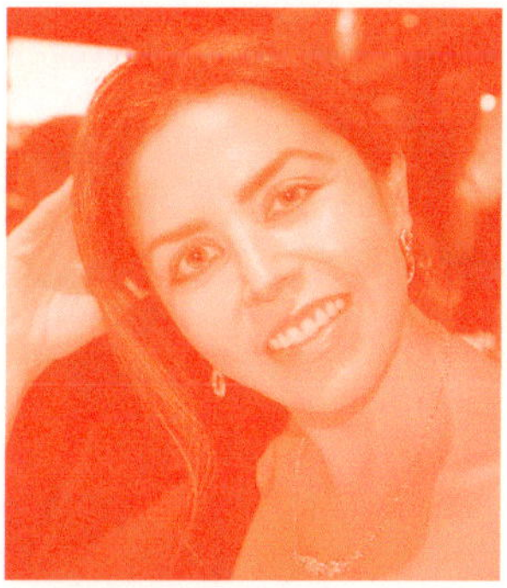

Supporting open minds since 2005

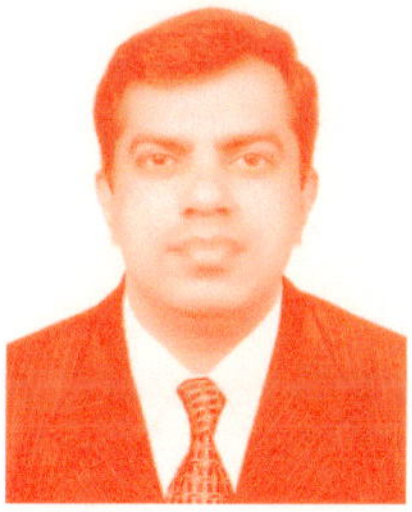
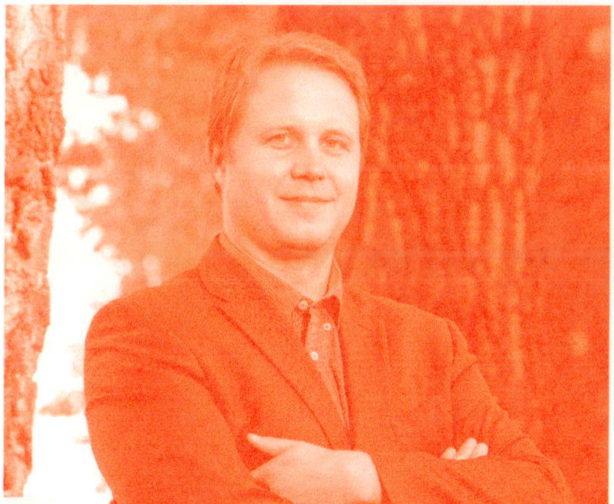
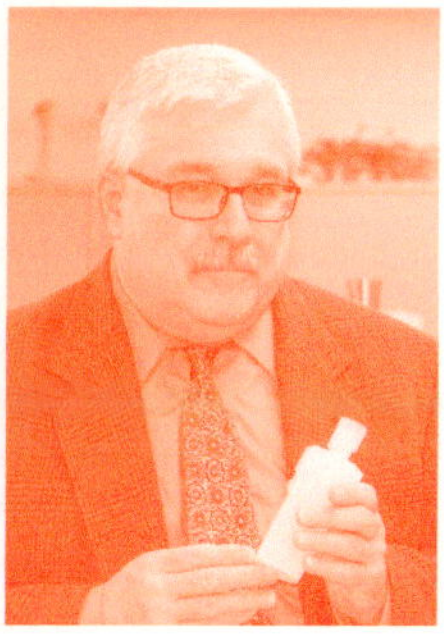
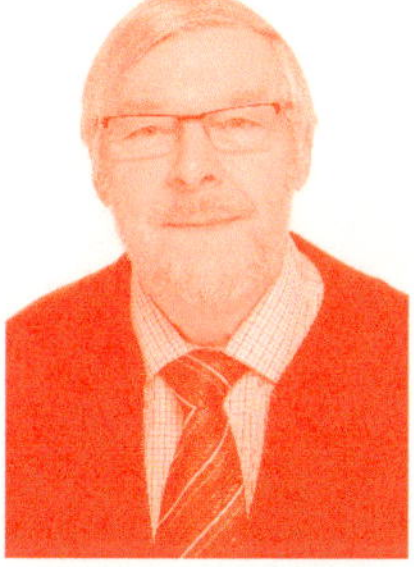
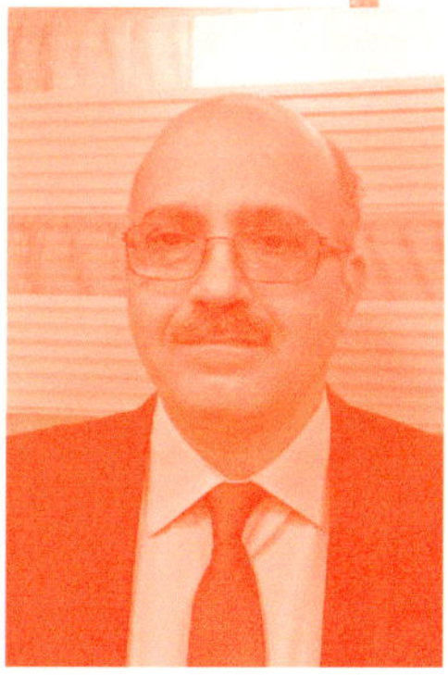
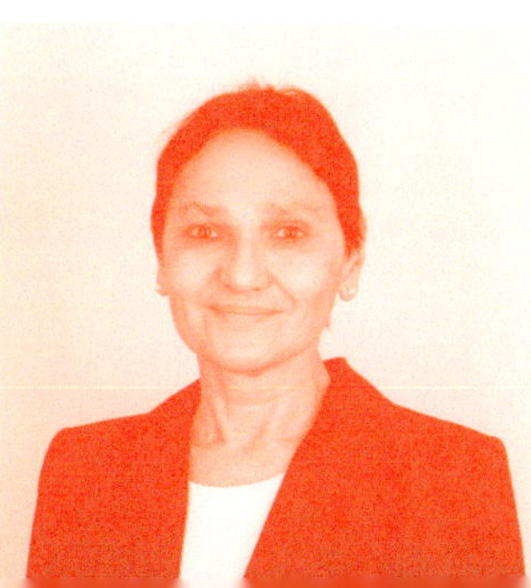
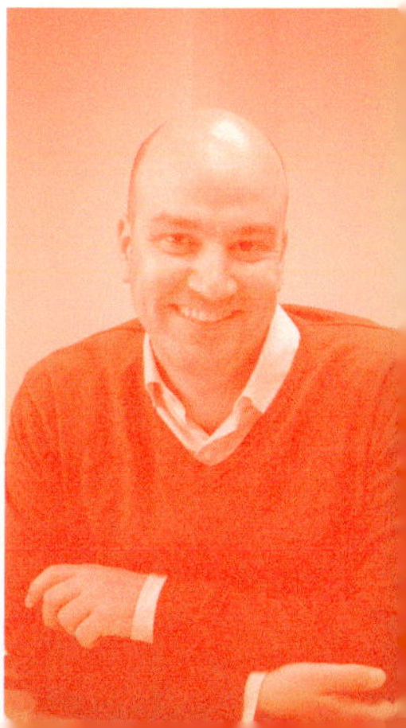

Essentials in Hip and Ankle
http://dx.doi.org/10.5772/intechopen.85454
Edited by Carlos Suarez-Ahedo, Anell Olivos-Meza and Arie M. Rijke

Contributors
Sachin Kumar Sharma, Hemant Mathur, Adinun Apivatgaroon, Nefiss Mouadh, Ben Maatoug Aymen, Teborbi Anis, Tekaya Asma, Ezzaouia Khelil, Bouzidi Ramzi, Naomi Kobayashi, Shota Higashihira, Yutaka Inaba, Tarcísio Santos Moreira, Yanyu Chen, Rachana Dabadghav

First published in London, United Kingdom, 2020 by IntechOpen
IntechOpen is the global imprint of INTECHOPEN LIMITED, registered in England and Wales, registration number: 11086078, 7th floor, 10 Lower Thames Street, London, EC3R 6AF, United Kingdom
Printed in Croatia

British Library Cataloguing-in-Publication Data
A catalogue record for this book is available from the British Library

Additional hard and PDF copies can be obtained from orders@intechopen.com

Essentials in Hip and Ankle
Edited by Carlos Suarez-Ahedo, Anell Olivos-Meza and Arie M. Rijke
p. cm.
Print ISBN 978-1-83880-325-4
Online ISBN 978-1-83880-326-1
eBook (PDF) ISBN 978-1-83962-601-2

For EU product safety concerns:
IN TECH d.o.o., Prolaz Marije Krucifikse Kozulić 3, 51000 Rijeka, Croatia, info@intechopen.com or visit our website at intechopen.com.

Meet the editors

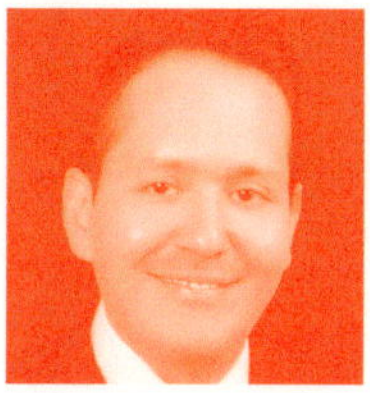

Dr. Suarez-Ahedo is a recognized orthopedic surgeon leading minimally invasive total hip and total knee replacement, sports medicine and arthroscopic surgery, providing superior knowledge and expertise to his patients. Dr. Suarez-Ahedo regularly gives lectures and teaches courses for orthoaedic surgeons around the world and is actively involved in the research and development of new techniques in joint replacement and arthroscopic surgery. He is also author and coauthor of several scientific publications in recognized international journals in the field of sports medicine, arthroscopic surgery, and hip pathology. Dr. Suarez-Ahedo is a La Salle University graduate (Mexico). He completed his training in Orthopedic Surgery at the Spanish Hospital in Mexico City. His subspecialty training includes a fellowship in Articular Surgery, fellowship in Adult Joint Hip and Knee Reconstruction at the National Rehabilitation Institute of Mexico, and an additional Fellowship in Hip Preservation Surgery at the American Hip Institute in Chicago, USA. His professional affiliations include International Member of the American Academy of Orthopaedic Surgeons (AAOS), the Arthroscopy Association of North America (AANA), and the International Society of Technology in Arthroplasty (ISTA), the International Society for Hip Arthroscopy (ISHA), and the Société Internationale de Chirurgie Orthopédique et de Traumatologie (SICOT).

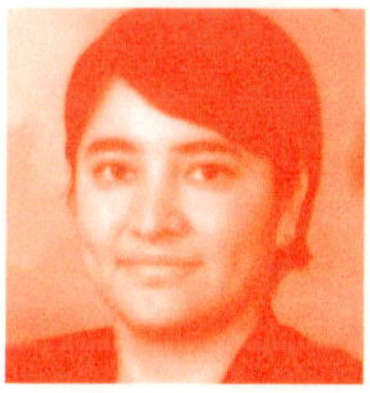

Dr. Anell Olivos-Meza graduated from Universidad Veracruzana, Xalapa Veracruz, Mexico in 2004, and completed her internship at the National Institute of Medical Science and Nutrition "Salvador Zubiran", Mexico City from 2004 to 2005. Dr. Olivos-Meza received her Medical Degree in 2007 from the University of Veracruz. She has been a Research Fellow in the Cartilage and Connective Tissue Laboratory (2007-2008) at Mayo Clinic College of Medicine, Rochester Minnesota, USA. In 2010, she completed her Master's degree in clinical research at the University of Veracruz. From 2011 until 2012 she was a part of the Direction and Administration of Medical Units (Postgraduate Studies) at the University of Puebla (Benemérita Universidad Autónoma de Puebla), Puebla, Mexico. Dr. Olivos-Meza completed the Orthopedic Surgery Residence Program from 2008-2012 at the Center of Medical Specialties in Veracruz State "Dr. Rafael Lucio", Xalapa, Veracruz, Mexico. From 2012 until 2013 she attended a Low Limb Articular Surgery Fellowship Program at the National Institute of Rehabilitation, Mexico City. She was a Clinical Visitor in the Low Limb Adult Reconstruction Service, Mayo Clinic, Rochester, USA, on several occasions in 2012. In 2014 she completed the Orthopedic Sports Medicine and Arthroscopy Fellowship Program at the National Institute of Rehabilitation. Mexico City. Her PhD Program was in the field of cartilage repair (2012-2016) at the Universidad Nacional Autónoma de México (UNAM) and National Institute of Rehabilitation, Mexico City. She is a member of several societies, such as: International Cartilage Repair & Joint Reconstruction Society; Mexican Orthopedic Society; Orthopedic Research Society Global Engagement Committee; Research Committee at the Instituto Nacional de Rehabilitación; Ethic Committee at the Instituto Nacional de Rehabilitación.

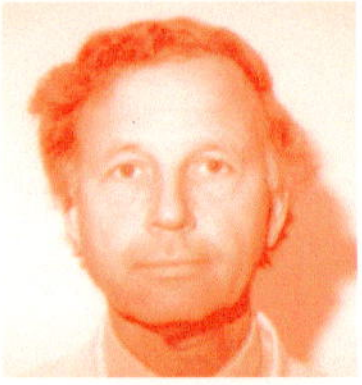
Arie M. Rijke has a Ph.D degree in physical chemistry and an M.D. degree specializing in musculo-skeletal radiology. He has held faculty positions in the School of Medicine and the School of Engineering of the University of Virginia since 1970. He is the Founder and President of Sport Tech, Inc., a company that specializes in diagnostic equipment for the evaluation of injury to the clinically important ligaments of the ankle, knee, shoulder, and elbow. The company uses its patent rights in the manufacture of the LigMaster product.

Contents

Preface

This book is intended to provide a concise, yet comprehensive introduction to some common hip and ankle pathologies and their treatment. Newer concepts continue to evolve and to keep abreast with these one should have a sound basic knowledge of the subject.

Every attempt has been made to narrate the concepts in a simplified manner keeping the originality. Wherever possible illustrations have been used to help the reader to understand the subject. The target audience comprises orthopedic surgeons, either in practice or in training, as well as clinicians, radiologists, and physical therapists.

The text is divided into two sections with short chapters providing a broad overview of the anatomy, pathology, and treatment. Selected references are also provided without the claim of being exhaustive and with the aim of stimulating interest and discussion.

We hope that we have succeeded in providing a useful and practical tool for the identification of some hip and ankle pathologies, and we remain open to any suggestions and criticisms for improvement in the future.

Carlos Suarez-Ahedo
Hospital Medica Sur,
Mexico City

Anell Olivos-Meza
Instituto Nacional de Rehabilitación,
Mexico

Arie M. Rijke
University of Virginia,
USA

Section 1

Hip

Chapter 1

Surgical Anatomy of Acetabulum and Biomechanics

Sachin Kumar Sharma and Hemant Mathur

Abstract

Both column acetabular fractures are challenging articular injuries. Majority of them are treated operatively. The concept of "secondary congruence" was introduced by Letournel. Despite this, biomechanical data on secondary congruence indicate that nonoperative treatment leads to an increase in peak pressures in the supra-acetabular region with the potential risk of developing posttraumatic degenerative osteoarthritis. Operative management is therefore justified. A cohort of 10 patients having both column (anterior and posterior) acetabular fractures managed using bicolumnar plating between Jan 2016 and Dec 2017 were enrolled in the study and were analyzed during follow-up period. Eighty percent of the patients had excellent to good result. Average postoperative score was 85.7. Assessment was done using Modified Harris Hip score.

Keywords: anterior and posterior column fracture, modified Harris Hip score, corona mortis, secondary congruence

1. Introduction

Hip arthroscopy requires a thorough knowledge of acetabular and pelvic anatomy. Acetabular and pelvic anatomy is complex yet important for any procedure to be done on hip joint. The articular surface of acetabulum can be visualized as being supported between the limbs of an inverted "Y". These two limbs are considered anterior and posterior columns of acetabulum. On radiographic view, anterior column is represented by iliopectineal line and posterior column by ilioischial line. Discontinuity in any of these lines is considered fracture of anterior or posterior column. The external iliac and internal iliac arteries lie in close relation to these columns. An anomalous connection of these two arteries called circle of death or corona mortis should be identified and ligated properly as injury to this artery can lead to catastrophic results. Lumbar plexus and its various nerve roots traverses the lesser and greater sciatic notches and are vulnerable to injury in portal placement and various other hip surgeries. This chapter mainly focuses on various aspects of surgical anatomy of acetabulum and biomechanics relevant to hip arthroscopy in detail.

2. Surgical and applied anatomy of the acetabulum

Treatment of acetabular fractures requires a deep understanding of pelvic anatomy. With advent of various minimally invasive approaches and fixation methods, knowledge of acetabular anatomy plays a pivotal role in treatment of displaced acetabular fractures. This chapter focuses on various aspects of acetabular anatomy, which are very vital in acetabular fracture fixation and also in other pelvic surgeries [1–5].

2.1 Osseous anatomy

The pelvis is the bony structure that transmits the weight of the upper axial skeleton to both the lower extremities via hip joint [1–5]. It comprises of the sacrum and three bones on each side that coalesce during adolescence to form the innominate bone of the adult pelvis. The iliosacral joint connects the sacrum to ilium. The ilium becomes the pubis anteriorly and the ischium inferiorly. Two pubic bones are connected to one another via the symphysis.

2.1.1 Acetabulum

The three bones, the ilium, ischium and pubis, join each other centrally to form the acetabular cavity. The blood supply to the femoral head traverses through the cotyloid fossa and ligamentum teres in childhood. The horse shoe-shaped cartilaginous portion of acetabulum is the main region through which the weight is transmitted from lower limb to innominate bone [4–6].

2.1.1.1 Column concept of the acetabulum

The acetabulum is an incomplete hemispherical socket with an inverted horse shoe-shaped articular surface surrounding the nonarticular cotyloid fossa. Two columns of bone which form an inverted 'Y', form and support the cotyloid fossa anteriorly and posteriorly [6–8] (**Figure 1**).

The anterior half of the iliac crest, the iliac spines, the anterior half of the acetabulum and the pubis form the anterior column.

The ischium, the ischial spine, the posterior half of the acetabulum and the dense bone forming the sciatic notch form the posterior column.

The shorter posterior column meets with the anterior column at the top of the sciatic notch. The column concept is very vital not only for classification of acetabular fractures but also in deciding the operative approach and hence the management. The weight-bearing portion of the articular surface is known as the dome or roof that supports the femoral head. The goal of both operative and nonoperative treatment is the anatomic restoration of roof or dome with concentric reduction of femoral head [8–10] (**Figure 2**).

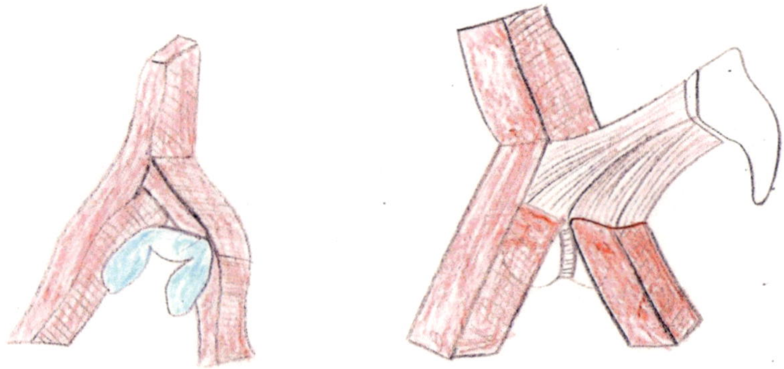

Figure 1.
Column concept of the acetabulum by Letournel and Judet.

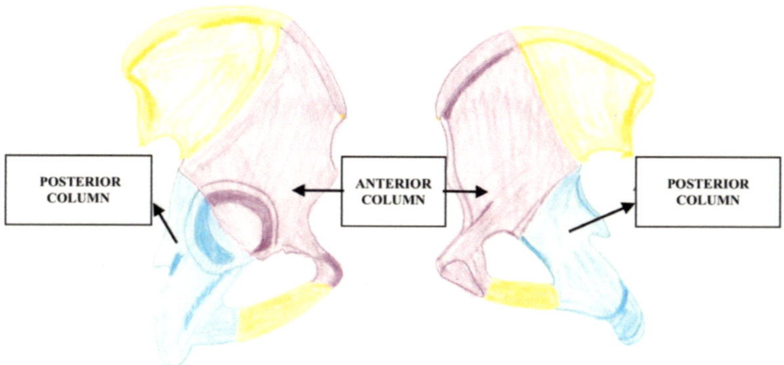

Figure 2.
Anterior column and posterior column.

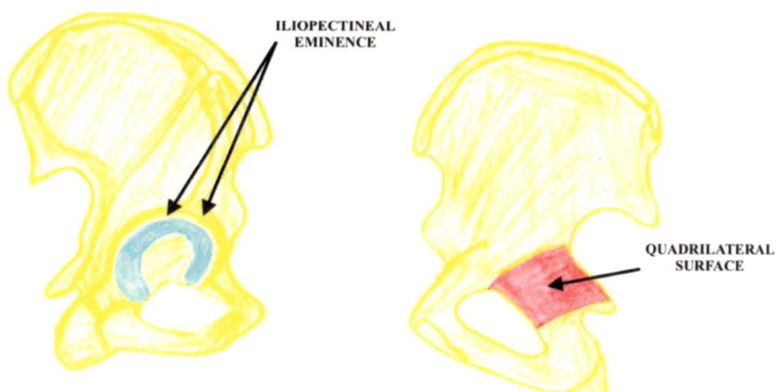

Figure 3.
Quadrilateral surface and iliopectineal eminence.

The flat plate of bone forming the lateral border of true pelvic cavity is known as quadrilateral surface. It lies adjacent to the medial wall of the acetabulum. The iliopectineal eminence is the prominence in the anterior column that lies directly over the femoral head. Both these structures limit the fixation of anterior column fractures of acetabulum [10] (**Figure 3**).

2.1.2 Iliac wing and innominate bone

The external iliac fossa is marked with two semi-circular lines dividing it into three zones [1–5]:

- Posterior (gluteus maximus)
- Middle (gluteus medius)
- Anterior (gluteus minimus)

Looking from above iliac wing appears S shaped. It begins anteriorly with a slight medial oblique orientation. Posteriorly it forms posterior iliac spine which is sagittally oriented. The iliac wing contains hematopoietic and osteogenic marrow elements and is the primary source of autogenous bone graft. Various structures are attached on different sides of iliac crest. The lower extremity hip motors are attached on the outer side. Along the inner portions, the iliacus and obturator internus and the pelvic floor musculatures are attached. The abdominal (anteriorly) and paraspinal (posteriorly) muscles are attached on the top [11, 12].

There is a strong buttress of bone extending from the iliosacral joint toward the acetabulum known as the sciatic buttress. The lumbosacral plexus as well as the gluteal vasculature lies in the vicinity. These vessels are the main source of bleeding and they can also be injured during surgical approach. The posterior superior iliac spine is adjacent to the sacroiliac joint and outer ilium.

The neurovascular structures exit the pelvis along with the piriformis muscle through sciatic notch. Sacrospinous ligament, the gemellus superior and the levator ani are inserted on the ischial spine. On the inferior side of ischial spine is the lesser sciatic notch, which contains the obturator internus tendon. The pudendal vessels and nerves pass through this area first exiting the pelvis via grater sciatic notch and then re-entering the pelvis via lesser sciatic notch.

The anterior-most border of the iliac bone begins with the anterosuperior iliac spine (ASIS), which gives origin to:

- Fascia Lata
- Sartorius
- Inguinal ligament

The antero-inferior iliac spine (AIIS) lies just below the ASIS where the *direct head of the rectus femoris* is inserted. The *iliopsoas muscle* passes just medial to AIIS under which lies the iliopectineal eminence. Indirect head of the rectus femoris is attached inferior to AIIS.

The boundaries of obturator foramen is formed by the pubis superiorly, the ischium inferiorly, and the anterior horn of the acetabulum posteriorly. Medially, the ischial and pubic rami join to form the symphyseal pubic junction. At its supero-lateral border, the obturator duct is present, which is occupied by obturator vessels and nerve. Obturator membrane covers the foramen circumferentially, which is a thick fascial structure. The integrity of the inguinal ligament and obturator membrane prevents the separation of rami fractures during reduction and fixation of symphyseal plate.

2.2 Ligament anatomy: the joints

The iliosacral joint is a fibrocartilaginous joint that acts as a dual wedge in axial and antero-posterior directions [12–15]. It acts as a keystone during the transmission of force to the lower limbs. The joint is supported anteriorly and posteriorly by strong ligaments. The posterior sacroiliac ligament consists of

- The superficial part going from the posterior iliac crest and posterior iliac spines to the posterior tubercles of the sacrum made up of several fascicles.
- The deep portion or interosseous ligament, which is the strongest ligament in the human body.

The sacrotuberous ligament connects sacrum to the ischial tuberosity (**Figure 4**).

The sacrospinous ligament connects the border of sacrum and coccyx and sciatic spine deep to sacrotuberous ligament. This ligament divides the ischial area into two foramens:

i. The Greater Sciatic Foramen: contains the piriformis muscle, superior glutei nerves, sciatic nerve, ischial vessels, and internal pudendal vessels and nerve.

ii. The Lesser Sciatic Foramen: contains the obturator internus muscle and internal pudendal vessels. These structures exit the pelvis via greater sciatic foramen and after crossing over the sacrospinous ligament re-enters the pelvis via lesser sciatic foramen [13–15].

2.3 Vascular anatomy

The aorta bifurcates in the lower peritoneal region into the common iliac arteries. The common iliac artery is begins at around L4 and divides at around the L5–S1 junction into the external and internal iliac arteries.

The internal iliac artery also known as hypogastric artery, branches to form the superior and inferior gluteal vessels, the obturator, the pudendal, and the coccygeal, the sacral and vesicular vessels. The internal pudendal artery exits the pelvis underneath the piriformis and re-enters the pelvis through the lesser sciatic notch and terminates as the dorsal artery of the penis and clitoris and cavernous artery [16, 17].

The external iliac artery just proximal to the inguinal ligament branches to form the femoral artery.

The femoral artery has three rami: urethral inferior, epigastric and iliac circumflex. The epigastric travels deep and then anastomoses with obturator vessels. The corona

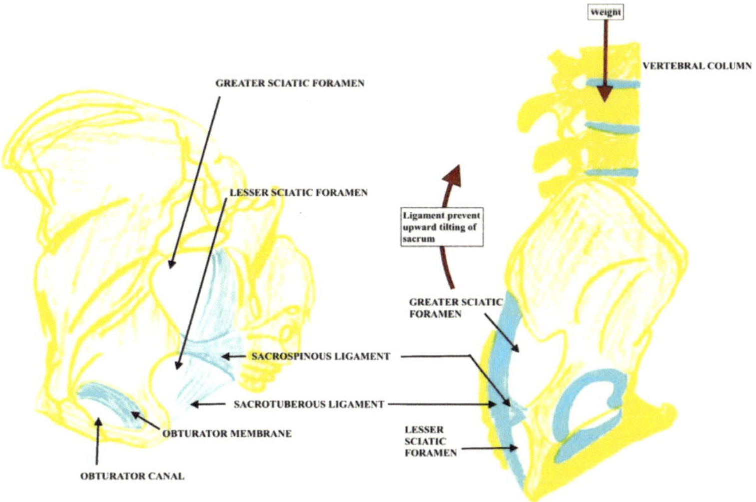

Figure 4.
The sacrotuberous and sacrotuberous ligaments.

mortis is the anomalous connection between epigastric and obturator vessels. It can cause fatal bleeding if not identified and ligated during surgery [17, 18] (**Figure 5**).

2.4 Neurologic anatomy

There are two important plexus: lumbar plexus and sacral plexus.

The Lumbar plexus consists of the first three lumbar anterior rami and a portion of the anterior ramus of the fourth lumbar nerve. There are also short collateral rami, which include the hypogastric, ilioinguinal, genitofemoral, and lateral femoral cutaneous nerve. Femoral and obturator nerves are the terminal rami of lumbar plexus.

The obturator nerve receives contributions from the L2, L3, and L4 trunks. It continues into the pelvis underneath the iliopectineal line, reaches the obturator orifice. It exits the pelvis together with the obturator vessels.

The femoral nerve receives contributions from the L2, L3, and L4 trunks [19–21].

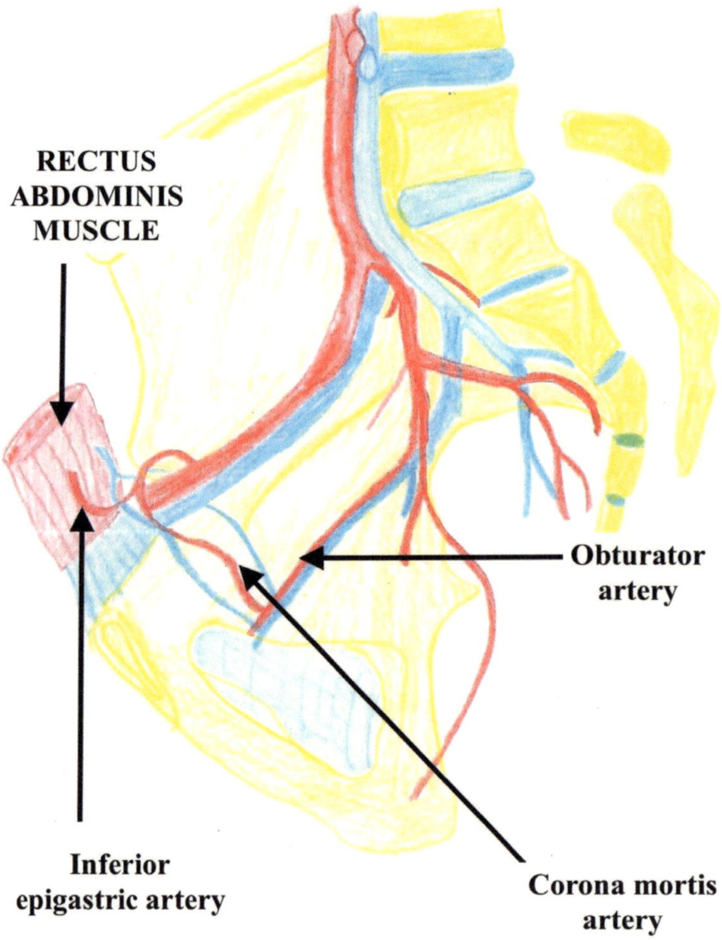

Figure 5.
Corona mortis artery.

The Sacral Plexus is formed by the coalescence of the lumbosacral trunk (L5 anterior ramus with L4 anastomotic ramus) and the anterior rami of the first four sacral roots. The plexus ultimately becomes the sciatic nerve (posterior tibial and peroneal nerve). The posterior branches relevant to orthopedic surgery are the superior gluteal nerve, branches to the external rotators and inferior gluteal nerve. The sciatic nerve exits the greater sciatic notch. In 85% of the cases, it courses in front of the piriformis. The other variants include penetration and splitting around the muscle. After exiting through greater sciatic notch, it courses behind the obturator internus, under the gluteal sling to enter the thigh. The sciatic nerve is a vital structure that is encountered during posterior approaches to the acetabulum. Due to proximity of sciatic nerve and its branches to the posterior part of acetabulum, fractures and dislocations in this area have very high incidence of sciatic nerve injury. Most common to be involved is the peroneal division of sciatic nerve [21, 22] (**Figure 6**).

3. Radiographic evaluation

The classification and subsequent treatment of acetabular fractures are based on imaging studies that have been derived from a thorough understanding of the

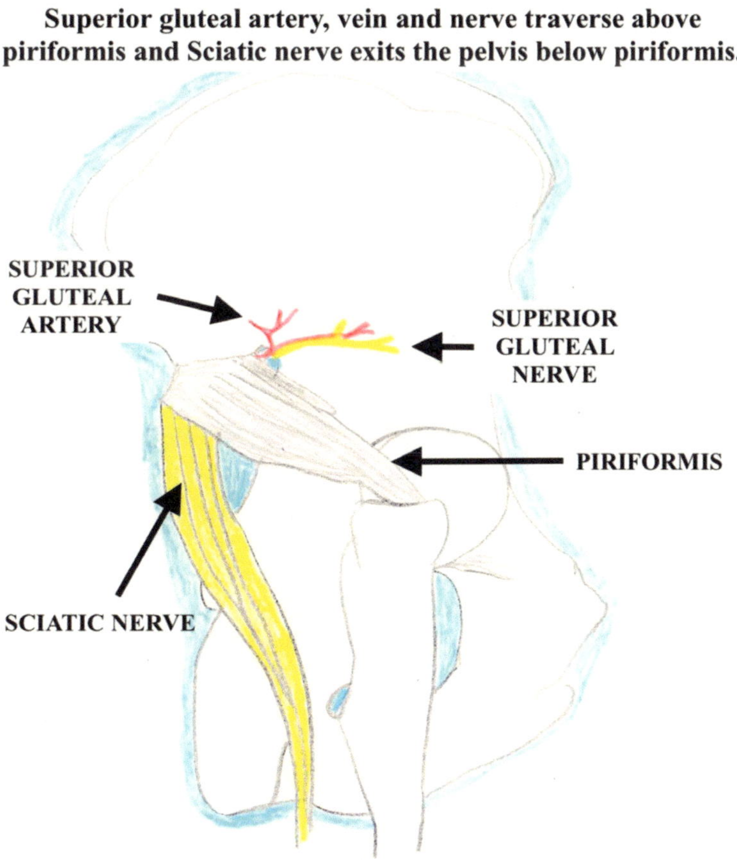

Figure 6.
The greater sciatic notch is divided by the piriformis.

anatomy of the innominate bone [17–19]. Two limbs of an inverted "*Y*" of bone support the articular surface of acetabulum. These columns are connected to the sacroiliac articulation by a thick strut of bone lying above the greater sciatic notch known as the sciatic buttress.

The radiographic anatomy of the acetabulum can be determined using AP pelvis and two 45-degree oblique radiographs as proposed by Judet and Letournel. Therefore, three radiographic projections of the pelvis that are used to evaluate the fractures of acetabulum are as follows:

- The antero-posterior view of the pelvis
- The obturator (or 45-degree internal, Judet) oblique view
- The iliac (or 45-degree external, Judet) oblique view

These plain films are interpreted based on the understanding of normal radiographic landmarks of the acetabulum, and disruption of these landmarks represents a fracture involving that portion of the bone. These landmarks are referred to as "lines". They are generated by the tangency of the applied x-ray beam to a region of cortical bone.

3.1 Antero-posterior radiograph

There are six basic landmarks (**Figure** 7)

- Iliopectineal line
- The ilioischial line
- The radiographic teardrop
- The roof of the acetabulum
- The anterior rim of the acetabulum
- The posterior rim of the acetabulum

The Iliopectineal Line is the major landmark of the anterior column. The pelvic brim is represented by anterior three-quarters of the iliopectineal line. The posterior quarter of this line is formed by the tangency of the x-ray beam to the internal cortical surface of the sciatic buttress and the internal part of the roof of the greater sciatic notch.

The Ilioischial Line is considered a radiographic landmark of the posterior column. It is formed by the tangency of the x-ray beam to the posterior portion of the quadrilateral surface.

The Radiographic Tear drop is not a true anatomic structure. It represents a radiographic finding and consists of a medial and lateral limb. The lateral limb represents the inferior aspect of the anterior wall in the acetabulum whereas the medial limb is formed by the obturator canal and the antero inferior portion of the quadrilateral surface. Dissociation of the teardrop and the ilioischial line indicates a fracture of the quadrilateral surface.

The Roof of the Acetabulum is a radiographic landmark that results from the tangency of the x-ray beam to a narrow portion of the subchondral bone of the superior acetabulum. Dissociation of the radiographic line of the roof indicates a fracture involving the superior acetabulum.

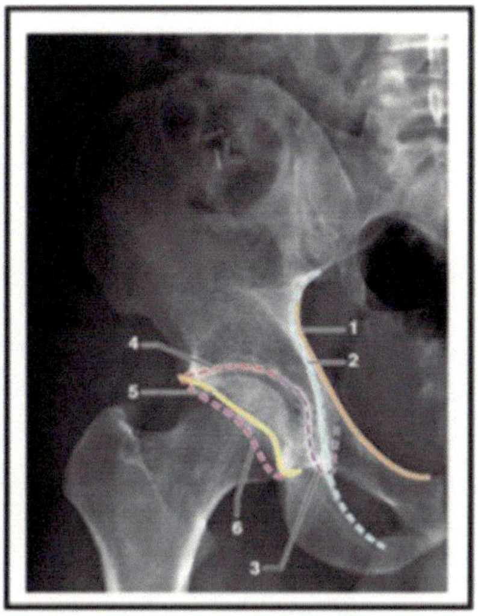

1. Iliopectineal line
2. Ilioischial line
3. Radiographic tear drop
4. Roof of acetabulum
5. Edge of anterior lip of acetabulum
6. Edge of posterior lip of acetabulum

Figure 7.
Radiographic landmarks on AP radiograph of hip.

The Anterior Rim of the Acetabulum represents the lateral margin in the anterior wall of the acetabulum and is contiguous with the inferior margin of the superior pubic ramus. The anterior rim is typically medial to the posterior rim and has a characteristic undulation in its midcontour in the AP pelvis view.

The Posterior Rim of the Acetabulum represents a lateral margin in the posterior wall of the acetabulum. Inferiorly, the posterior rim is contiguous with the thickened condensation of the posterior horn of the acetabulum and approximates a straight line, being more vertical than the anterior wall.

3.2 The iliac oblique view (also known as external oblique view)

This view is obtained by rotating the patient so that the injured hemipelvis is tilted 45 degrees away from the x-ray beam. Structures visible on this view are greater and lesser sciatic notches, anterior rim of acetabulum and iliac wing in its largest dimension. This is the best view to see the fractures involving posterior column. Fractures of the anterior column traversing the iliac wing can also be detected.

3.3 The obturator oblique view (also known as internal oblique view)

This view is obtained by rotating the patient so that the injured hemipelvis is rotated 45 degrees toward the x-ray beam. This view shows the obturator foramen in its largest dimension and profiles the anterior column. The posterior rim of the acetabulum is best visualized in the obturator oblique view.

Posterior subluxation of femoral head can be detected by comparing the relationship of the femoral head with the posterior wall on the normal hip and the injured hip on the obturator oblique view. A dislocated hip will become more obvious in the obturator oblique view, and this view has been advocated for routine evaluation of all posterior fracture dislocations of the hip joint. It is prudent not to delay the reduction of a known dislocated hip (**Figure 8**).

Dynamic stress views under general anesthesia have also been used in acetabular fractures. They serve as a clinical measure of dynamic stability and congruence of

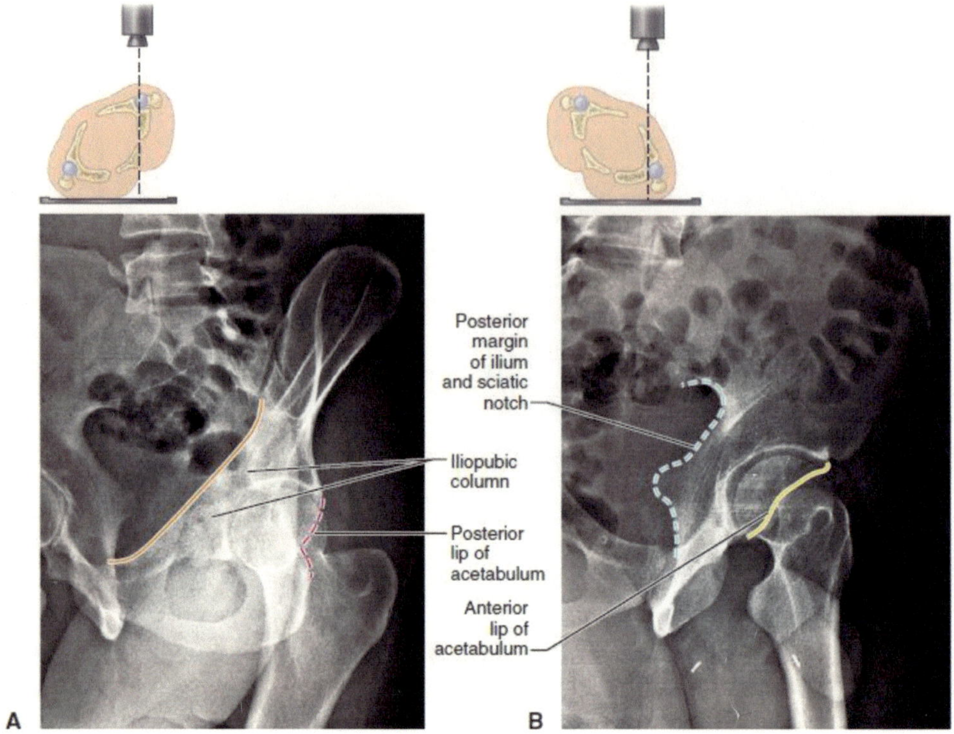

Figure 8.
(A) obturator oblique view and (B) iliac oblique view.

X-ray view	Information regarding
Antero-posterior pelvis	
Iliopectineal line	Anterior column
Ilioischial line	Posterior column
Posterior lip	Posterior column or wall
Anterior lip	Anterior column or wall
Roof	Superior articular surface
Teardrop	Relationship of columns
Obturator oblique	
Pelvic brim	Anterior column
Posterior rim	Posterior column or wall
Obturator ring	Column involvement
Roof	Superior articular surface
Iliac oblique	
Greater and lesser sciatic notch	Posterior column (posterior border of innominate bone)
Quadrilateral surface of ischium	Posterior column (posterior border of innominate bone)
Anterior lip	Anterior column or wall
Iliac wing	Anterior column
Roof	Superior articular surface

Table 1.
Information obtained from X-ray landmarks on each standard view [17–19].

the hip thus helps in assessing the need for operative treatment in small and intermediate fractures of the posterior acetabular wall. This stress examination is most applicable to the fractures of posterior wall.

Each fracture pattern in the classification of Letournel and Judet has typical radiographic characteristics. These fracture patterns are described with respect to the disruption or intactness of the radiographic landmarks.

In the operating room, the three standard views can be obtained with fluoroscopy. The restoration of the radiographic landmarks marks the adequacy of fracture reduction (**Table 1**).

4. Computed tomography

CT plays a pivotal role in the treatment of acetabular fractures [18, 19]. Axial cuts should be taken with thin (3-mm) intervals and corresponding slice thicknesses. To avoid missing a portion of the fracture the entire pelvis is generally included and comparison to the opposite hip is performed routinely. In general, the transverse fracture lines and fractures of the anterior and posterior walls are in the sagittal plane, paralleling the quadrilateral surface when they are viewed on axial CT images.

Some authors have suggested that axial CT images overestimate the extent of comminution of acetabular fractures. An oblique fracture line divides the acetabulum, so the more inferior CT cuts appear to have three fragments when in reality there are only two. By studying the individual fragments on multiple successive cuts, the entire fracture can be appreciated, giving a true mental three-dimensional picture. High-resolution coronal and sagittal reconstructions of the fracture are helpful in the preoperative evaluation of complex fractures by delineating the fracture lines that lie directly in the plane of a given axial CT image.

CT scans can give the same information about the acetabular dome as the roof arc measurements on the antero-posterior and oblique radiographs.

Three-dimensional CT reconstructions of a fracture have become sophisticated and can be projected in many different views with the subtraction of the femoral head that show unique features of the various fracture patterns [16] (**Figure 9**).

4.1 Role of 3D CT in acetabular fractures

The late 1970s and early 1980s saw the development of software and hardware that made it possible to produce 3D reformats of complex anatomical structures from sets of transaxial CT images [19]. However, the acceptance of 3D was limited because of poor image quality, lack of user-friendly systems, and limited display flexibility. In past few years, several manufacturers have introduced software that is easier to use and that produces 3D views much faster than the earlier systems. Several investigators now believe that the spatial analysis of a complex acetabular fracture is best made with 3D imaging. Some investigators have stated that 3D CT is a valuable addition to the imaging of acetabular fractures.

The original transaxial slices show the diagnostic details, but 3D imaging integrates the finding into a whole that is more easily assimilated than the sum of its parts. By having an access to a 3D image, the surgeon can decide whether or not to operate and which approach to use. Although 3D images may present less detail to the radiologist than the 2D series, but for an operating surgeon 3D images are very helpful for re orientation during surgical repair. Minor non-displaced fractures are unlikely to require or benefit from 3D reformats [23–26] (**Figure 10**).

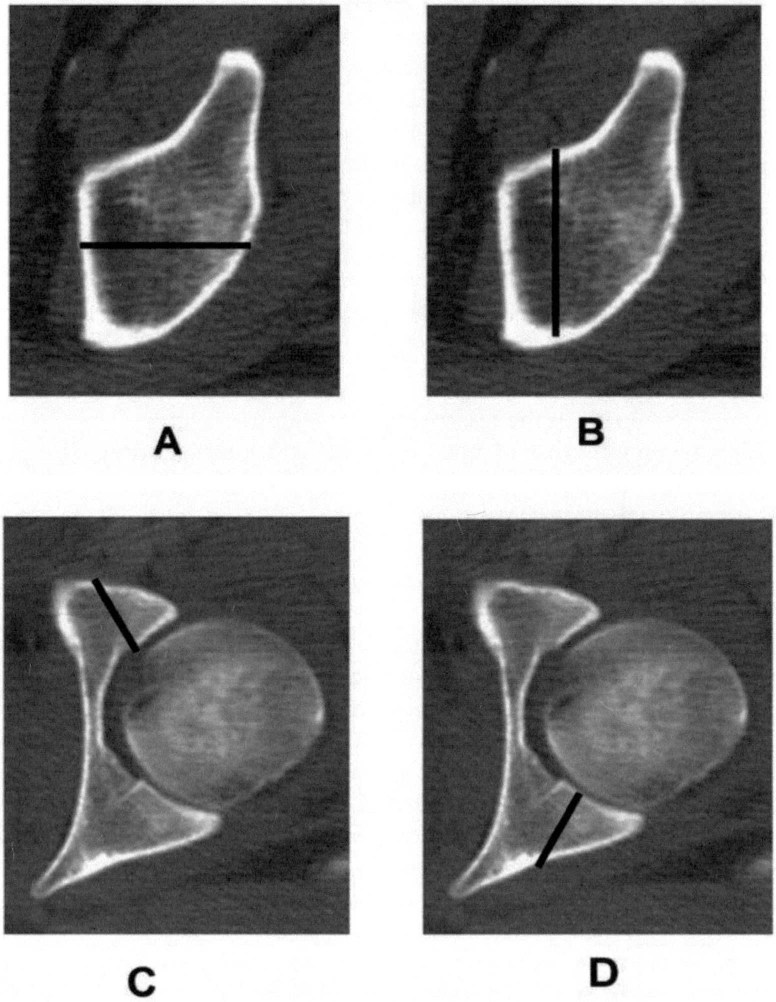

Figure 9.
Orientation of fracture lines on two-dimensional computed tomography as they relate to fracture morphology. (A) Fracture of one or both columns. (B) Transverse fracture. (C) Anterior wall. (D) Posterior wall.

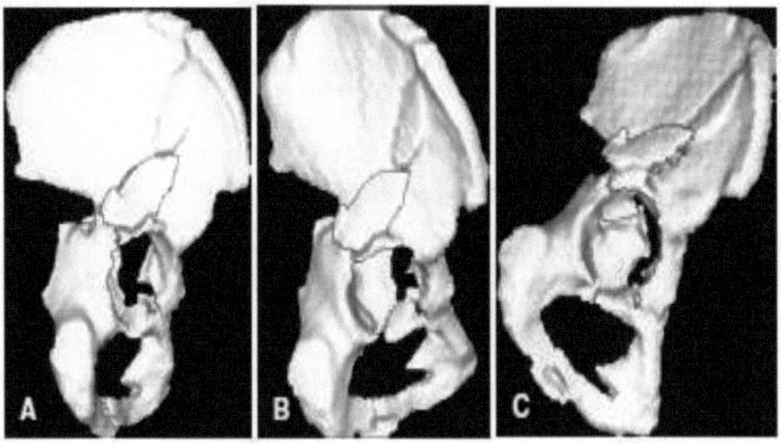

Figure 10.
Three-dimensional CT reconstruction of both-column fracture.

5. Classification

Classification of acetabular fractures is the key element in understanding the injury and is the first stage of surgical planning [17, 18]. Decisions concerning the choice of approach and the alternative fixation techniques available require full appreciation of the fracture anatomy. There are various classifications for acetabular fractures, out of them Letournel and Judet and AO/OTA classification has been discussed in detail here.

5.1 Letournel and Judet classification

The classification of acetabular fractures that is most widely used is that of Letournel and Judet. This system divides fracture of acetabulum into five simple (elementary) and five complex (associated) patterns. The elementary fracture patterns were defined as those that separated all or parts of a single column of the acetabulum. The associated patterns are either a combination of elementary patterns with an additional fracture line (**Figures 11** and **12**).

Elementary/simple fractures

- Posterior wall
- Posterior column
- Anterior wall
- Anterior column

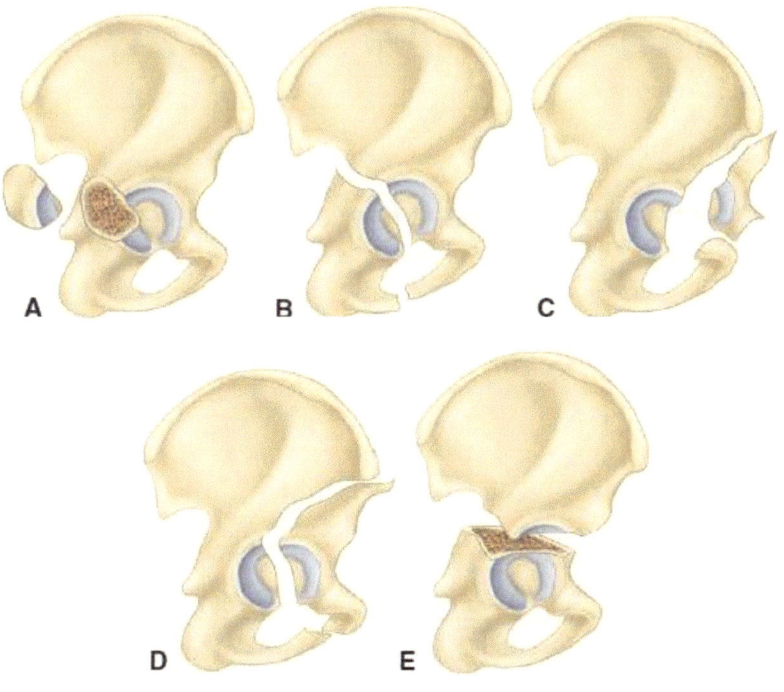

Figure 11.
Simple/elementary fractures: (A) posterior wall fracture, (B) posterior column fracture, (C) anterior wall fracture, (D) anterior column fracture, (E) transverse fracture.

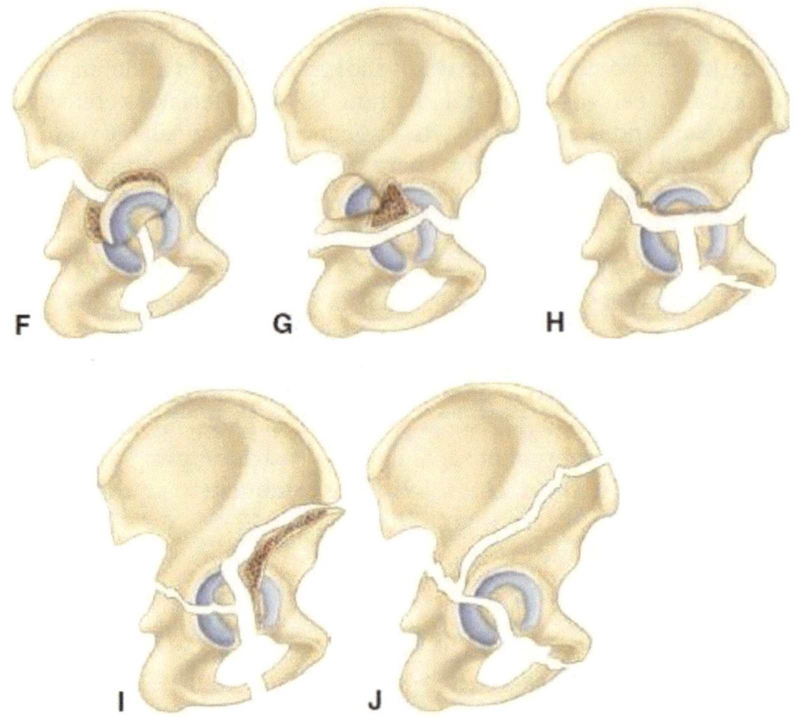

Figure 12.
Associated fractures: (F) Posterior column and posterior wall fracture, (G) Transverse and posterior wall fracture, (H) T-shaped fracture, (I) Anterior column and posterior hemitransverse fracture (J) Complete both column fracture.

- Transverse

Associated fractures

- Posterior column + wall
- Anterior + posterior hemitransverse
- Transverse + posterior wall
- T-shaped
- Both columns

6. Surgical approach for each fracture pattern

One of the most important aspect of the preoperative planning for acetabular fracture surgery is the selection of appropriate surgical approach [23, 24]. The main determinants in the decision-making process are the type of fracture, the elapsed time from injury to operative intervention, and the magnitude and location of maximal fracture displacement. The mainstay surgical approaches to the acetabulum are those described by Letournel and Judet (**Table 2**):

Fracture pattern	Approach
Elementary	
Posterior wall	Kocher-Langenbeck
Posterior column	Kocher-Langenbeck
Anterior wall	Ilioinguinal or iliofemoral
Anterior column	Ilioinguinal or iliofemoral
Transverse	Kocher-Langenbeck or ilioinguinal
Associated	
Posterior column + posterior wall	Kocher-Langenbeck
Anterior column + posterior hemitransverse	Ilioinguinal
Transverse + posterior wall	Extended iliofemoral or Kocher-Langenbeck
T-shaped	Extended iliofemoral or combined
Both columns	Ilioinguinal or extended iliofemoral or combined

Table 2.
Surgical approaches used for various fracture patterns.

- The Kocher-Langenbeck
- The ilioinguinal
- The iliofemoral
- The extended iliofemoral

6.1 Modified Stoppa approach

General agreement exists for the use of the modified Stoppa approach for all fractures that can be managed with an ilioinguinal approach [24]. This includes anterior wall, anterior column, and associated anterior column and posterior hemi transverse fractures, as well as certain both- column, T-shaped, and transverse fractures. The Stoppa approach is particularly useful for fractures that involve the quadrilateral surface with or without comminution and medial dislocation of the femoral head.

7. Biomechanics of the acetabulum and applied mechanics of fracture fixation

7.1 Normal mechanics of the hip joint

Of the many joints in the human body, the hip joint has been the one which has attracted the most attention from investigators [26, 27]. The reasons are; first, in normal activity this joint carries the greatest load, load intensity fluctuating between zero and its maximum during each cycle of activity; secondly, probably because of this loading, mechanical failures of the hip joint and of the neighboring bony structure, particularly the upper femoral region, constitute a large proportion of the problems confronting the orthopedic surgeon.

Mechanical forces acting within the normal hip joint are complex and difficult to quantify precisely. During locomotion, large forces occur across the hip joint in which each leg alternately supports the weight of the body. During mid-stance, little acceleration and relatively constant force are applied across the joint, making midstance ideal for a static loading model of investigation. Forces across the joint itself are greatest during midstance and are derived from two primary sources:

- Body weight (BW)

- Abductor moment (Abd)

Body weight is centered just anterior to S2 vertebra and exerts a force on the hip joint, which acts to rotate the pelvis about the femoral head toward the center of gravity. Counteracting this force is the *abductor moment*, this act to rotate the pelvis in the opposite direction. During single-leg stance, these two forces cancel each other out and, therefore, the pelvis remains upright.

Because both of these forces have magnitude and direction, they can be expressed as vectors on a free body diagram. The Abd is greater than BW, owing to a shorter moment arm, so that in the steady state.

$$(\text{BW} \times a) = (\text{Abd} \times b)^2 \qquad (1)$$

The joint reactive force is the compressive force experienced at the femoroacetabular articulation, and it is the result of the need to balance the moment arms of the body weight with the pull of the hip abductors at the greater trochanter to maintain a level pelvis (**Figure 13**).

The primary contributions to the joint reactive force are the muscular forces generated to level the pelvis during standing and gait, with a smaller contribution from body weight. The magnitude of this force varies with activities such as the single leg stance phase of gait and it has been found to be as much as 2–4 times the body weight during level walking and stair ascent and slightly higher during stair descent [27, 28].

Smooth gait relies on a well-synchronized series of concentric and eccentric muscular contractions to facilitate a balanced stride. A complete neuromuscular loop exists that maintains the appropriate position between the femoral head and acetabulum with balanced muscular regulation achieved at both the voluntary and involuntary level.

The weight-bearing portion of the hip has been found to vary with position of the femur in relation to the acetabulum and the amount of load placed through the articulation. During normal loading of a nonarthritic joint during activities such as walking, majority of the articular surface participates in weight bearing. This involves the anterior, superior and posterior parts of the femoral head and forms two columns of force that are transmitted within the acetabular margin, joining at the superior aspect of the acetabular fossa. The geometric orientation of the articular cartilage is also optimized for load transfer, because the thickest portions are at the areas of the acetabulum and femoral head most frequently loaded during gait.

7.2 Biomechanical consequences of acetabular fracture

A number of studies have focused on the biomechanical consequences of acetabular fracture [28–32]. These studies can be divided into those focusing on.

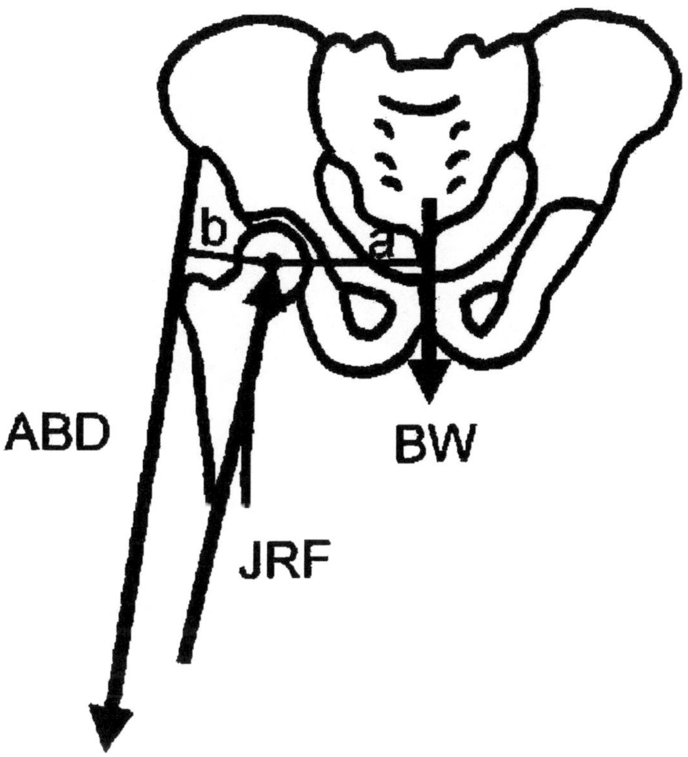

Figure 13.
*A line drawing of hip joint loading. The joint reaction force vector of the hip is the result of the moments around the hip caused by two opposing surface. The **body weight (BW)** is centered in front of S2 and is distance **away** from the center of the femoral head. The **force of the abductor muscle (Abd)**, centered from the midiliac wing to the greater trochanter is distance **b** away from the femoral head. During single-leg stance, the product of BW × distance a will equal the force of the Abd × distance b. Because distance b is much shorter than a, the force of the abductor mechanism is greater.*

1. Intra-articular contact area and pressure.

2. Rigidity of fracture fixation.

3. Instability or loss of congruence after fracture.

The studies that focus on contact area and pressures argue that increased joint stress from incongruity or altered loading characteristics eventually will lead to degenerative posttraumatic arthritis through repetitive cartilage damage. The guiding hypothesis is that increased stresses within the cartilage exceed the capacity of the tissue to adapt, initiating a cascade of degenerative changes that ultimately leads to arthritis in the joint. It showed that increased peak pressures, especially in the superior region of the acetabulum, do lead to degenerative arthritis.

Clinically, attempts to define the weight-bearing portion of the acetabulum have used *the roof arc measurement*, which represents the angle formed between a vertical line drawn to the geometric center of the acetabulum and a tangential line drawn from the geometric center to the point at which the fracture line enters the joint on antero-posterior and Judet view radiographs. When measured on standard antero-posterior and 45° oblique radiographs, the roof arc measurement gives an estimation of the amount of articular surface remaining intact (**Figure 14**).

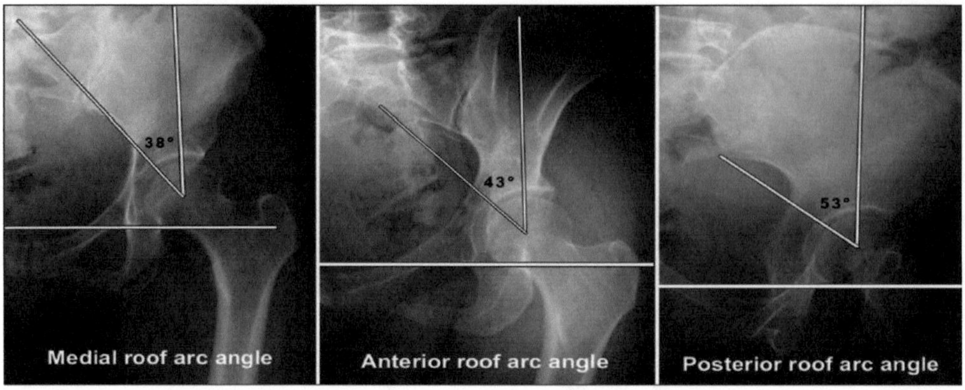

Figure 14.
Medial, anterior and posterior roof arc angle.

7.2.1 Intra-articular contact characteristics

Several studies have focused on the alteration of contact area and stresses in the joint as a result of the fracture [28–32]. All fracture patterns showed a change from a uniform contact pattern to one of increased contact area and peak pressures in the superior acetabulum.

Letournal introduced the concept of "secondary congruence" in both column fractures of the acetabulum. In this group, the complete separation of all articular acetabular bony fragments can lead to an extra anatomical orientation around the femoral head with the possibility of healing in secondary congruence. In contrast, Levine et al. found an increase of the mean pressure and peak pressure in the acetabular roof area, whereas the contact area and mean pressure between femoral head and acetabular surface was decreased significantly in the anterior articular region and on a lesser degree in the posterior region.

8. Significance of surgical anatomy in hip arthroscopy

Surgical anatomy plays a pivotal role in hip arthroscopy as erroneous placement of portals can lead to injury to various important structures as described previously in the chapter. A surgeon should be well aware of various landmarks as well as vital structures around the hip joint while making portals and also while working through these portals.

One of the disastrous complication of hip arthroscopy is injury to sciatic nerve or femoral nerve and vessels. Various evidences suggest that these injuries can be prevented when proper technique in portal placement was used.

Another structure that is quite often injured during hip arthroscopy id lateral femoral cutaneous nerve of thigh (LFCN). LFCN is mostly injured during anterior portal placement. Injury to this nerve leads to loss of sensation on lateral aspect of thigh. The nerve is essentially vulnerable to laceration by a skin incision placed too deeply through the subcutaneous tissue.

Apart from these, if proper surgical anatomy is known, injury to various soft tissues around hip can also be minimized considerably. It is prudent for the surgeon to be aware of various anatomical structures around hip then only a safe and successful surgery can be performed.

9. Conclusion

Anatomy has always been a second wife for a surgeon. Its role cannot be neglected whether it is a minor or major surgery. When it comes to advanced surgeries like arthroscopy requiring meticulous techniques, surgical anatomy becomes more important. If a surgeon is well versed with surgical anatomy, many iatrogenic injuries can be avoided considerably.

Conflict of interest

None.

Source of funding

Self.

Author details

Sachin Kumar Sharma* and Hemant Mathur
Government Medical College and SSG Hospital Vadodara, Gujarat, India

*Address all correspondence to: docsachinsharma0@gmail.com

References

[1] Eichenhiltz SN, Stark RM. Central acetabular fractures. Journal of Bone and Joint Surgery. American Volume. 1964;**46A**:4

[2] Beaule PE, Dorey FJ, Matta JM. Letournal classification of acetabular fractures. Journal of Bone and Joint Surgery. American Volume. 2003;**85A**:9

[3] Stewart MJ. Discussion of prognosis of fractures of acetabulum. Journal of Bone and Joint Surgery. American Volume. 1961;**43A**:59

[4] Laird A, Keating JF. Acetabular fractures: A 16 year prospective epidemiological study. Journal of Bone and Joint Surgery. British Volume. 2005;**87**:969-973

[5] Muller ME et al. Manual of Internal Fixation. Berlin Heidelberg: Springer-Verlag; 1992

[6] Matta J. Fractures of the acetabulum: Accuracy of reduction and clinical results in patients managed operatively within three weeks after the injury. Journal of Bone and Joint Surgery. American Volume. 1996;**78A**:1632-1645

[7] Kleinberg S. Fracture of acetabulum with central luxation of the hip. Annals of Surgery. 1923;**78**(6):806-813

[8] Olson SA. Diagnosis and Treatment of Acetabular Fractures: Historic Review. 1st ed. USA: Informa Healthcare; 2007

[9] Bircher M. Pelvic and acetabular fractures past, present and future. AO Dialogue. 2007;**1**(07):36-39

[10] Rogers LF, Novy SB, Harris NF. Occult central fractures of the acetabulum. Journal of Bone and Joint Surgery. American Volume. 1975;**124**:1

[11] Bray TJ, Esser M, Fulkerson L. Osteotomy of the trochanter in open reduction and internal fixation of acetabular fractures. Journal of Bone and Joint Surgery. 1987;**69**(5):711-717

[12] Murphy D, Kaliszer M, Rice J, McElwain P. Outcome after acetabular fractures: Prognostic factors and their inter relationships. International Journal of Injury. 2003;**34**(7):512-517

[13] Im GI, Chung WS. Fractures of posterior wall of acetabulum: Treatment with cannulated screws. International Journal of Injury. 2003;**10**:031

[14] Berton M, Jessica C, McMicheal. Outcome of posterior wall fractures of acetabulum. Journal of Bone and Joint Surgery. 2007;**89-A**:6

[15] Manson T, Schmidt A. Acetabular fractures in elderly. Journal of Bone and Joint Surgery. 2016;**4**(10):e1

[16] Pesantez R, Ziran BH. Anatomy of Pelvis: Fractures of Pelvis and Acetabulum. 1st ed. USA: Informa Healthcare; 2007

[17] Canale ST. Campbells Operative Orthopaedics. 12th ed. Vol. 3. Philadelphia, PA: Elsevier Inc.; pp. 2741-2796

[18] Bucholez RW, Hechman JD, Court Brown CM. Rockwood and Green's Fractures in Adults. 7th ed. Philadelphia, PA: Lippincot Williams and Wilkins Co.; 2012

[19] Lawrence DA, Men K, Baumgertner M, Hamis AH. Acetabular fractures: Anatomic and clinical considerations. American Journal of Roentgenology. 2013;**201**:W425-W436

[20] Pierannunzii L, Fisher F, Tagliabue L. Acetabular both

column fractures: Essentials of operative management. Injury: International Journal of the Care of the Injured. 2010:1145-1149

[21] Romanes GJ. Cunninghams' Manual of Practical Anatomy. 15th ed. Vol. 1. Oxford Publications; 1986

[22] Jarrod Durkee N, Jacobson J, Jamadar D, Karunakar MA, Morag Y, Hayes C. Classification of commom acetabular fractures: Radiographic and CT appearances. American Journal of Roentgenology. 2006;**187**:915-925

[23] De Boer P, Buckley R, Hoppenfield S. Surgical Exposures in Orthopaedics: The Anatomic Approach. 4th ed. Lippincot Williams and Wilkins Co.; 2011

[24] Cutrera NJ, Pinkas D, Toro JB. Surgical approaches to the acetabulum and modification in techniques. Journal of American Academy of Orthopedic Surgeons. 2015;**23**:592-603

[25] Laurence M, Freeman AR, Swanson AV. Section of orthopaedics. Journal of Bone and Joint Surgery. American Volume. 1966;**59A**

[26] Tile M, Helfet D, Kellam J. Fractures of Pelvis and Acetabulam. 3rd ed. Lippincot Williams and Wilkins Co; 2003

[27] Bowman KF, Fox J, Sekiya JK. A clinically relevant review of hip biomechanics. The Journal of Arthroscopic and Related Surgery. 2010;**26**(8):1118-1129

[28] Gansslen A, Hildebrand F, Krettek C. Conservative treatment of acetabular both column fractures: Does the concept of secondary congruence work? Acta Chirurgiae Orthopaedicae. 2012;**79**:411-415

[29] Lei J, Dong P, Li Z. Biomechanical analysis of the fixation systems for anterior column and posterior hemitransverse acetabular fractures. Acta Orthopaedica et Traumatologica Turcica. 2017;**51**:248-253

[30] Giannoudis PV, Grotz MRW, Papakostidis C, Dinopoulos H. Operative treatment of displaced fractures of the acetabulum (a meta-analysis of 34 studies). Journal of Bone and Joint Surgery. British Volume. 2005;**87-B**:2-9

[31] Mardanpour K, Rahbar M, Rahbar M, Mardanpour N, Mardanpour S. Functional outcomes of traumatic complex acetabular fractures with open reduction and internal fixation (a study of 200 cases). Open Journal of Orthopedics. 2016;**6**:363-377

[32] Rahimi H, Gharahdaghi M, Parsa A, Assadian M. Surgical management of acetabular fractures (a study of 44 cases). Trauma Monthly. 2013;**18**(1):28-31

Chapter 2

Femoroacetabular Impingement: Anatomy and Pathogenesis

Nefiss Mouadh, Ben Maatoug Aymen, Teborbi Anis, Tekaya Asma, Ezzaouia Khelil and Bouzidi Ramzi

Abstract

Femoroacetabular impingement (FAI) is an often unrecognized hip disorder in young adults that can lead to early hip osteoarthritis and a decrease in sports performance. The diagnosis and treatment of this entity have rapidly evolved in recent years. Hip arthroscopy finds its place in the treatment of this conflict, and its indications are more and more frequent. The technical challenge of this operation involves a relatively long learning curve and a good knowledge of the hip anatomy in order to minimize the risk of complications and iatrogenic lesions. In addition to intra-articular structures of the hip joint, the anatomical structures that may be affected by the main and accessory arthroscopic approach are primarily the lateral femorocutaneous nerve, the lateral circumflex femoral artery, the medial circumflex femoral artery, and the circumflex superior iliac artery. A little further, 3–5 cm from the main portals, we must pay attention to the femoral nerve, the sciatic nerve, the superior gluteal nerve, the profunda femoris artery, the superficial femoral artery, and the common femoral artery. The pathogenesis of femoroacetabular impingement is not fully understood. The multifactorial origin is still relevant today. We have divided factors incriminated in the genesis of FAI into three groups.

Keywords: femoroacetabular, impingement, anatomy, pathogenesis, arthroscopy

1. Introduction

Femoroacetabular impingement (FAI) is a common cause of early hip osteoarthritis. Often underdiagnosed, this entity deserves a particular interest in orthopedic surgeons.

In some cases of FAI, the underlying structural abnormality is secondary to residual childhood hip disorders, such as Legg-Calvé-Perthes disease, slipped capital femoral epiphysis, and others. In other cases, there is no obvious history of previous hip pathology, and the impingement is referred to as primary FAI [1]. The exact description of this morphological anomaly and how it causes early hip osteoarthritis has been studied by Ganz in 2001 [2]. However, Smith Petersen and Stulberg have talked about this pathology several years before [3, 4].

Diagnosis has become easier and easier with new imaging techniques, but clinical suspicion remains essential before any exploration.

Arthroscopy is the most common surgical procedure for FAI involving acetabuloplasty, labral repair/debridement, and/or femoroplasty [5].

Nakano [6], in a systematic review published in 2017, reported a complication rate of 3.3% after hip arthroscopy, and potential complications include neurovascular injuries, chondral and labral injuries, muscle pain, and avascular necrosis of femoral head and even femoral neck fracture [6–8].

This chapter reviews the bony, muscular, and neurovascular anatomies of the hip joint with specific attention to structures of greatest relevance to FAI and hip arthroscopy.

2. Methods

This chapter is a descriptive study of FAI anatomy and pathogenesis.

Anatomy figures were drawn by us to explain some anatomical relationships as well as the pathogenesis of FAI. Other figures are photographs and radiographs of patients followed and treated at our university hospital.

Concerning the literature research, the data sources used in our manuscript were PubMed, MEDLINE, and ScienceDirect.

The search terms used were femoroacetabular impingement OR FAI, anatomy, pathogenesis, and hip arthroscopy.

All study types were included, including case reports and review articles. Studies referenced in the selected papers were retrieved individually.

3. Anatomy of FAI

The morphology of the proximal femur and acetabulum can vary significantly, which can have an important clinical relevance and impact on hip joint biomechanics. The detailed anatomy of the hip is well described in the manuals of anatomy. In FAI, two types of hip morphology have been described, namely, the cam type and the pincer type. These two types may exist separately or be associated within the same patient.

Thus, the isolated presence of either cam or pincer morphology is insufficient for a diagnosis of FAI syndrome. It is important to note that these morphologies are thought to be fairly common (around 30% of the general population) including in people without hip symptoms [9, 10].

3.1 Cam morphology

It describes a flattening or convexity of the femoral head neck junction [6] (**Figures 1, 2**).

This morphology is more common in men [10].

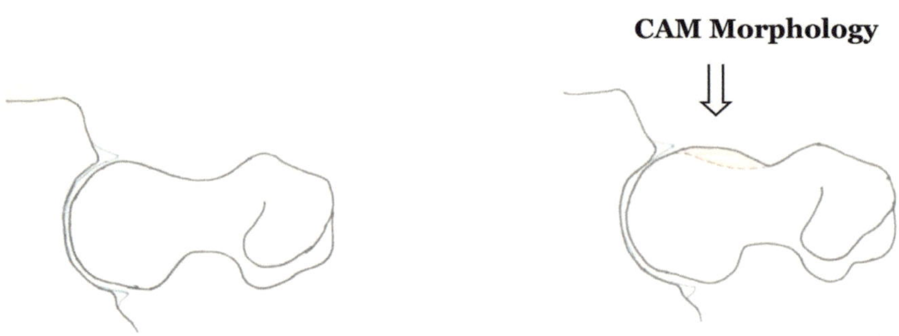

Figure 1.
Normal aspect of femoral head-neck junction versus cam morphology.

3.2 Pincer morphology

It describes the overcoverage of the femoral head by the acetabulum in which the acetabular rim is extended beyond the typical amount, either in one focal area or more generally across the acetabular rim [6] (**Figure 3**).

This morphology is more common in women [10].

These two types (CAM and Pincer Morphology) may exist separately or be associated within the same patient (**Figure 4**).

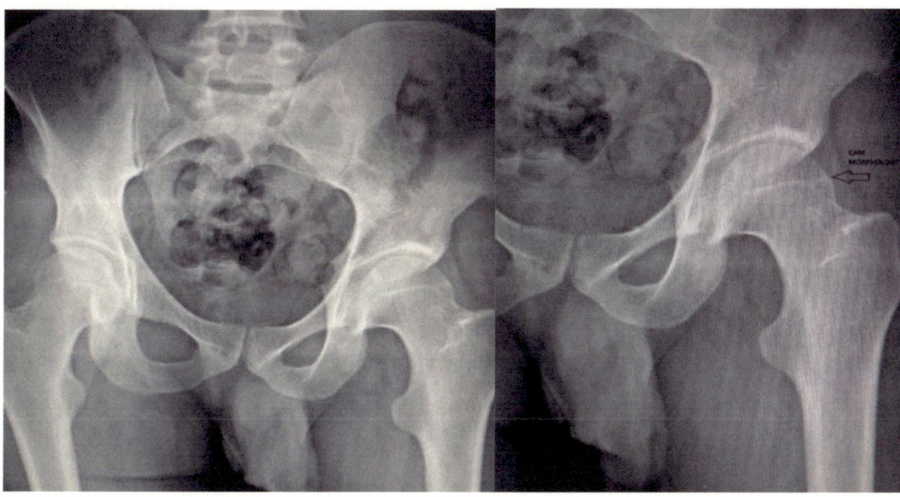

Figure 2.
CAM morphology in a young man with a childhood hip disease.

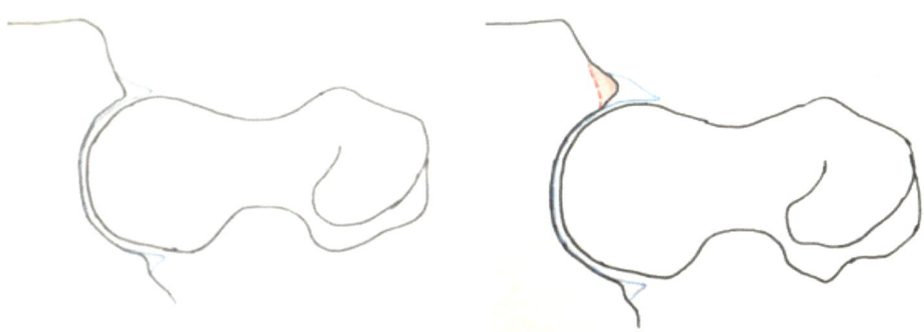

Figure 3.
Normal aspect of femoroacetabular junction versus Pincer morphology.

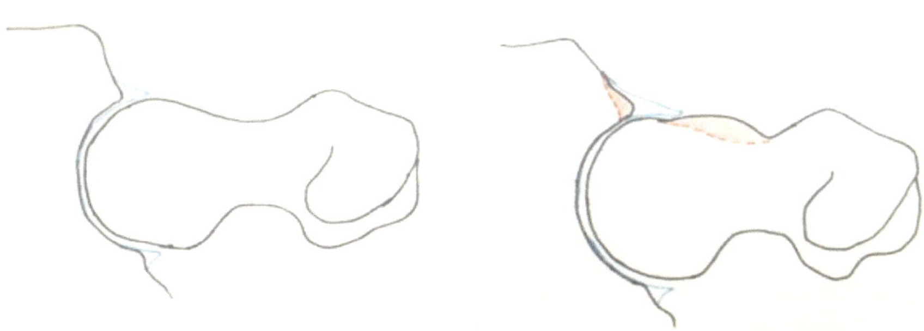

Figure 4.
Mixed morphology with both aspects of CAM and Pincer morphology.

Recently, several studies have shown that the prominence of the anterior-inferior iliac spine (AIIS) could also contribute to a conflict with the cervico-cephalic junction even if the hip anatomy is normal. This subspine impingement can simulate FAI and thus represents a differential diagnosis [11, 12].

3.3 Arthroscopic approach for FAI and anatomy of the hip

3.3.1 Superficial landmarks of the hip

Given the proximity of vasculo-nervous elements, identification of a so-called safe zone is essential in such a minimally invasive surgery requiring a good knowledge of hip region anatomy (**Figure 5**).

The identification of certain structures will depend on the degree of obesity of the patient.

The superficial landmarks conventionally used in hip arthroscopy for an FAI are the following.

3.3.1.1 The anterior-superior iliac spine (ASIS)

The hip being in neutral rotation, a vertical line joining the anterior-superficial iliac spine and the middle of the base of the patella forms the medial limit of the "safe zone." Beyond this line there is a higher risk of femoral nerve and femoral vessel injuries [13].

3.3.1.2 Great trochanter (GT)

Identification of the tip of the GT and its anterior and posterior edges is essential and easily felt. The anterolateral portal (AL) and the posterolateral portal (PL) are located 1 cm proximal and anterior or posterior to the tip of the GT, respectively. The

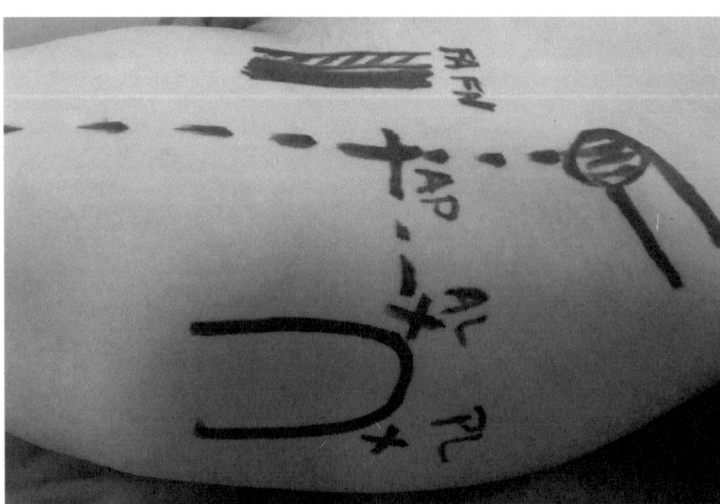

Figure 5.
Landmarks and main portal used in hip arthroscopy: PL, posterolateral portal; AL, anterolateral portal; AP, anterior portal; FA, common femoral artery; FN, femoral nerve.

anterior portal (AP) is located at the intersection of a transverse line passing through the AL and PL portals and a sagittal line drawn distally from the ASIS [13, 14].

3.3.1.3 Muscles

The muscles crossed during hip arthroscopy for a FAI are [14, 15]:

- The AP crosses the sartorius and then the rectus femoris. A more recent interpretation of AP is described as 1 cm laterally compared to the first marker, and it crosses tensor fascia latae before intersecting the interval between the gluteus minimus and rectus femoris.
- The AL portal crosses superficially the gluteal fascia at its junction with tensor fascia latae before deepening through the fibers of the gluteus medius muscle.
- The PL portal crosses the gluteal fascia and the gluteus medius; medially to the GT, it passes anterosuperiorly to the piriformis tendon before entering the lateral capsule in its posterior aspect.

3.3.2 Neurovascular structures

The vascular structures that need attention in hip surgery in general and in hip arthroscopy in particular are essentially the common femoral artery (CFA) and its two terminal branches, the profunda femoris artery (PFA) and the superficial femoral artery, (SFA) as well as three lateral branches, which are the circumflex superficial iliac artery (CSIA), the lateral circumflex femoral artery (LCFA), and the medial circumflex femoral artery (MCFA) (**Figure 6**).

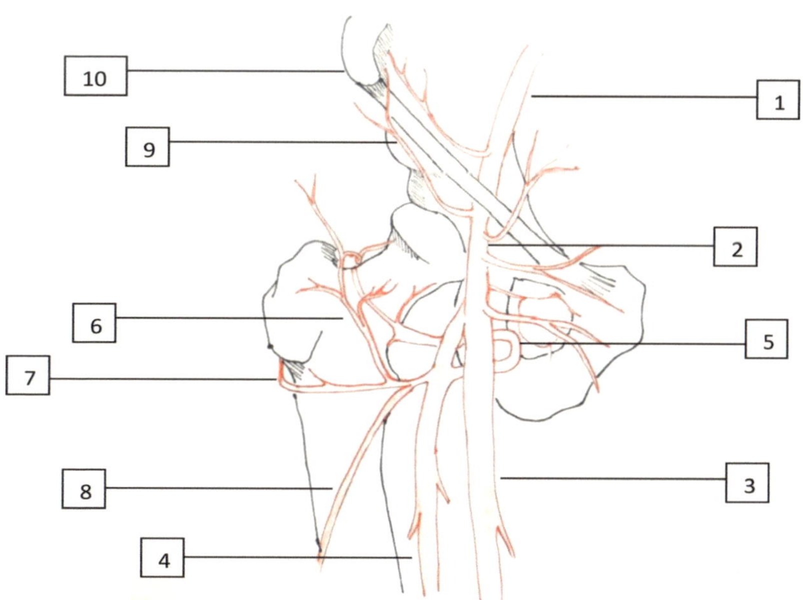

Figure 6.
Vessels to be considered in hip arthroscopy. (1) External iliac artery (EIA); (2) common femoral artery (CFA); (3) profunda femoris artery (PFA); (4) superior femoral artery (SFA); (5) medial circumflex femoral artery (MCFA); (6) lateral circumflex femoral artery (LCFA), ascending branch; (7) LCFA, transverse branch; (8) LCFA, descending branch; (9) circumflex superior iliac artery (CSIA); (10) anterior superior iliac spine (ASIS).

3.3.2.1 The common femoral artery

It continues the external iliac artery (EIA) and lies anterior and medial to the hip capsule. Only the iliopsoas lies between the vessel and capsule at this point, and it is continued by the superficial femoral artery. The femoral vein lies medial to the artery.

3.3.2.2 The circumflex superior iliac artery

A collateral branch of the CFA originates from its proximal part at the level of the Scarpa triangle and goes out toward the ASIS.

3.3.2.3 The profunda femoris artery

It lies medial to the SFA and continues the CFA 3 to 4 cm below the femoral triangle. It gives at the level of the hip the following collaterals.

3.3.2.4 The lateral circumflex femoral artery (LCFA)

It is a collateral branch of the PFA that originates from its proximal part (2–3 cm). It lies behind the sartorius and the rectus femoris and is divided into three branches:

- An ascending branch that vascularizes the GT and participates in the irrigation of the head and neck of the femur

- A transverse branch that passes through the large external muscle to anastomize with the MCFA

- A descendant branch that sometimes originates directly from the deep femoral artery and runs along the medial part of the vast outer back of the anterior right

The ascending branch of LCFA averaged 3.7 cm from the anterior portal. A terminal branch of this vessel was present in three specimens 0.3 cm from this portal [15] (**Figure** 7).

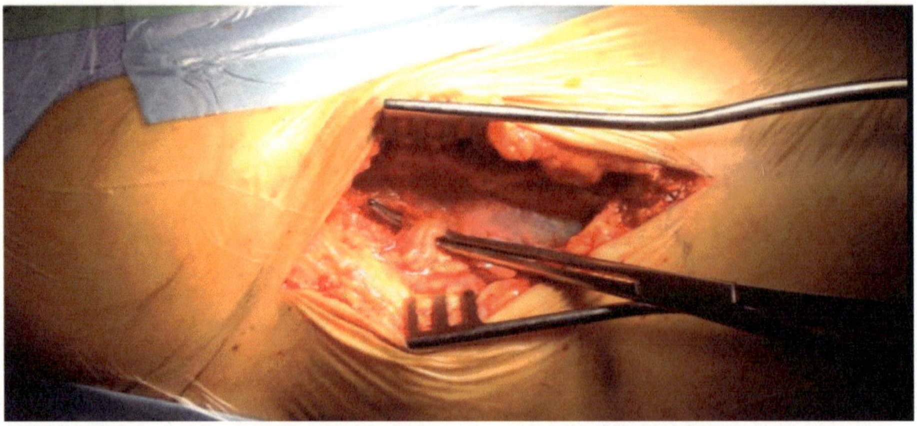

Figure 7.
Position and trajectory of the lateral circumflex femoral artery.

3.3.2.5 The medial circumflex femoral artery (MCFA)

It is a collateral branch of the PFA that originates 1–2 cm from its proximal part, journeys medially, and then wraps itself around the femoral diaphysis to give an ascending branch and a transverse branch that anastomoses with their counterparts of the LCFA.

Nerve structures that are at risk in hip arthroscopy are the femoral (FN), the sciatic nerve (SN), the lateral femorocutaneous nerve (LFCN), and the superior gluteal nerve (SGN).

3.3.2.6 The lateral femorocutaneous nerve (LFCN)

It emerges from underneath the inguinal ligament just medial to the ASIS and courses down along the surface of the sartorius muscle.

The proximal path of the nerve is relatively constant, but its branching is rather irregular, giving 0–5 branches when becoming more superficial; the most lateral of them are potentially on the course of AP (**Figures 8, 9**).

Byrd [14] in an anatomic study of portal placement and relationship to the extra-articular structures in hip arthroscopy found that the LFCN had divided into three or more branches at the level of the AP and that this portal averaged only 0.3 cm from one of these branches.

Larson and Clohisy [16, 17] in a prospective multicenter trial including 1505 hip arthroscopies and in systematic review found that the most common complication was postoperative LFCN disturbance (16.5%), which persisted beyond 6 months in only 1.6%.

3.3.2.7 The femoral nerve

The femoral nerve is the most lateral structure within the femoral triangle. It lies on the Psoas muscle belly at the approximate midpoint between the anterior superior iliac spine and pubic tubercle.

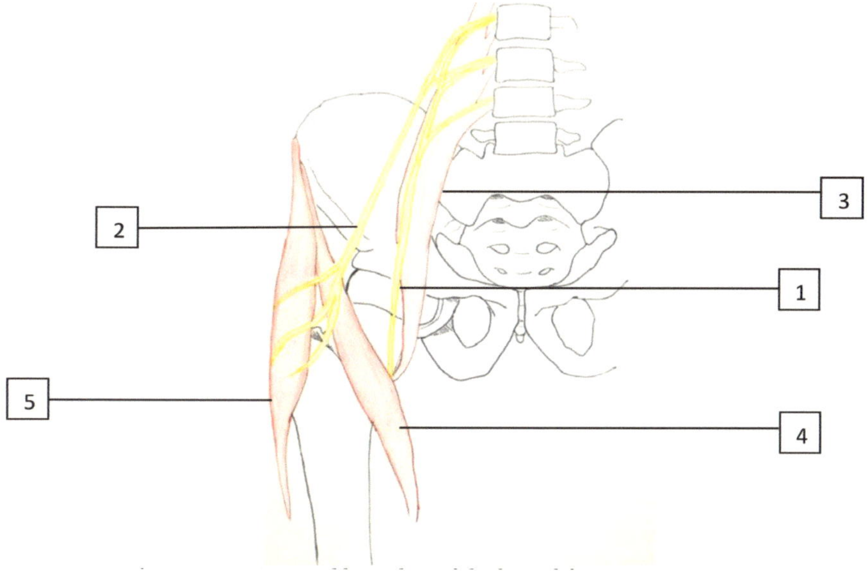

Figure 8.
Origin and branches of the lateral femorocutaneous nerve. (1) Femoral nerve; (2) lateral femorocutaneous nerve with its branch; (3) psoas muscle; (4) sartorius muscle; (5) tensor fascia latae muscle.

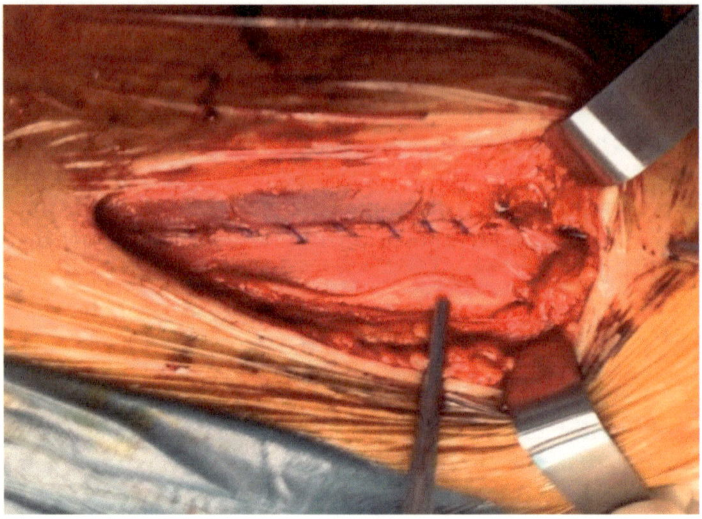

Figure 9.
A branch of the lateral femorocutaneous nerve accidentally cut in an anterior hip approach.

The average minimum distance from the anterior portal to the femoral nerve was 3.2 cm [15].

3.3.2.8 The sciatic nerve

The sciatic nerve averaged 2.9 cm from the poster lateral portal. From this study, these portal placements appear to be safe [15].

3.3.2.9 The superior gluteal nerve

It averaged 4.4 cm superior to the anterolateral and posterolateral portals [15].

Relations of these structures with arthroscopic portals have to be assessed and topographic knowledge of the delicate anatomy surrounding the hip fully understood [14].

4. Pathogenesis

The presence of a conflict between the acetabulum and the femoral head-neck junction was noted by several surgeons as being the cause of early hip osteoarthritis (**Figure 10**); however, it was Ganz [1] who was the first to describe details of FAI pathogenesis. He defined it as a condition of abnormal contact between femoral head-neck junction and the acetabulum due to abnormal morphological features and/or as a result of subjecting the hip to the excessive and supraphysiologic range of motion.

This repetitive contact causes a microtraumatic effect and subsequently irreversible chondral damage to the acetabular as well as femoral surfaces [18].

Based on a systematic review performed by Chaudhry and Ayeni, the etiology of FAI syndrome is likely multifactorial [4].

The main factors incriminated in the genesis of FAI belong to three groups:

- Factors related to the level and type of physical activity of the patient; indeed the FAI is particularly common among young athletes requiring extreme and repetitive movement of the hip in flexion and internal rotation such as hockey and basketball.
- Morphological abnormalities such as acetabular retroversion and coxa profunda or changes in hip morphology due to the history of childhood hip disease which may have altered the shape of the femoral head-neck junction such as slipped capital femoral epiphysis (SCFE) or Legg-Calvé -Perthes disease [4].
- Iatrogenic factors such as excessive correction of hip dysplasia or following an osteosynthesis of a neck or head fracture.

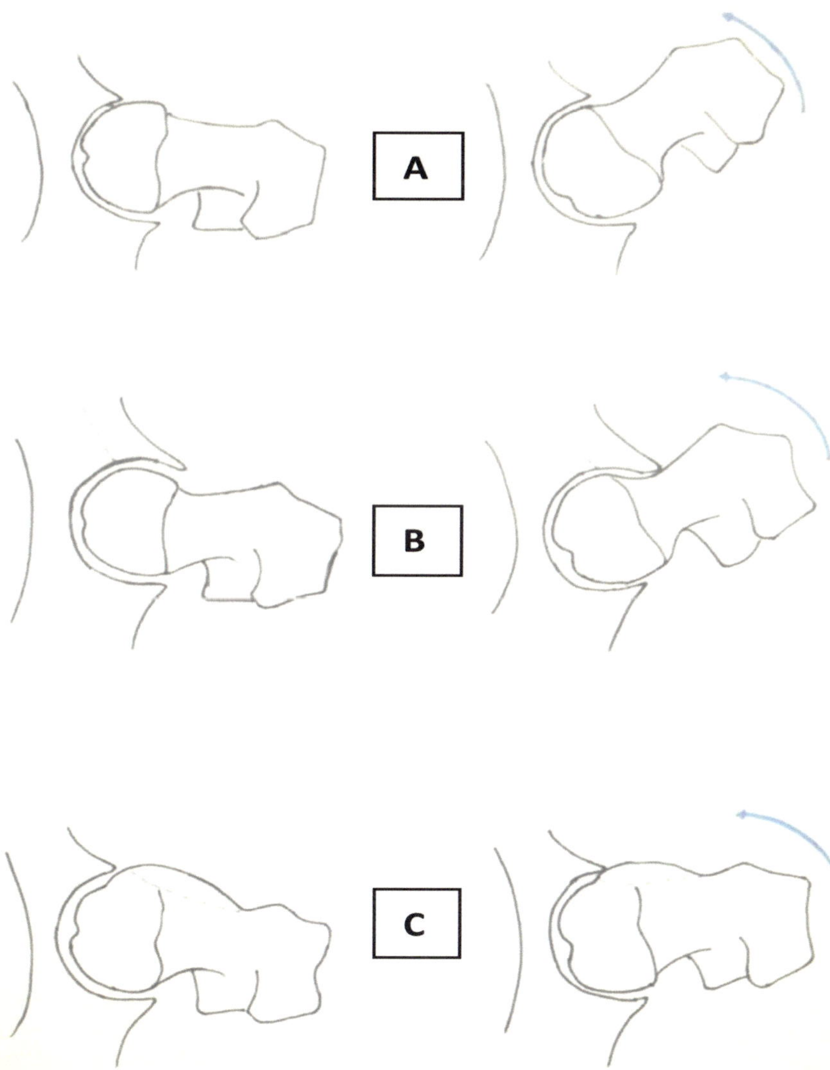

Figure 10.
Pathogenesis of femoroacetabular impingement. (A) Normal morphology; (B) mechanism of impingement in pincer morphology; (C) mechanism of impingement in cam morphology.

Given that cam and pincer morphologies can be present in asymptomatic individuals, Casartelli [19] propose that other factors out with the bony structures may be involved with FAI syndrome. Weakness of deep hip muscles could not only compromise hip stability but also lead to overload of secondary movers of the hip, thus causing an anterior glide of the femoral head into the acetabulum and increased joint loading.

5. Discussion

The hip region is an area where several noble elements pass including the femoral neurovascular bundle anteriorly, the LFCN anterolaterally, and the sciatic nerve and gluteal vessels posteriorly. Direct neurovascular injury is rare, except the LFNC; however, their proximity to portals and the effect of traction have to be considered by the surgeon especially during the learning curve.

In fact, during hip arthroscopy, a perineal post is used for countertraction and traction and is needed to provide space for instrument introduction which can lead to soft tissue injuries, and this is the most commonly reported complication of hip arthroscopy [20].

Risks and recommendation during hip arthroscopy and portals placement are detailed in **Table 1**.

	Risks	**Recommendations [20]**
Traction	1. Femoral and sciatic nerve neurapraxia 2. Pudendal nerve injury	1. Continuous traction should not exceed 2 hours The force of traction should be limited to <22.7 kg 2. Well-padded and wide enough perineal post
Anterior portal	1. Direct injury of the LFCN 2. Vascular injury (rare) 3. Iatrogenic labral and chondral injuries	1. Use lateralized anterior portal, and the skin incision should not extend into the subcutaneous fat 2. Optimal landmarks spotting and portal placement 3. Adequate traction (≥10 mm) Avoid repetitive exchange of instruments
Anterolateral portal	Iatrogenic labral and chondral injuries	Optimal portal placement
Posterior portal	Inferior gluteal artery and sciatic nerve injury (rare)	Optimal portal placement Avoid internal rotation of the hip while positioning this portal

Table 1.
Risks incurred during traction and portal placement.

6. Conclusion

FAI is explained by morphological abnormalities reaching the femoral head-neck junction or the acetabulum. Hip arthroscopy is widely used nowadays for its management.

To avoid complications of this technique, a good knowledge of hip anatomy is necessary as well as the risks incurred during its practice.

Traction and portal placement are the cause of most complications.

The lateral femorocutaneous nerve is the noble structure and the most exposed to injuries through the anterior portal. With the exception of it, direct major neurovascular injury is very rare; however, care is needed especially during the learning curve.

Author details

Nefiss Mouadh*, Ben Maatoug Aymen, Teborbi Anis, Tekaya Asma, Ezzaouia Khelil and Bouzidi Ramzi
Orthopedic Surgery Department, Faculty of Medicine, Mongi Slim Hospital, Tunis El Manar University, La Marsa, Tunisia

*Address all correspondence to: mouadhnefiss2@gmail.com

References

[1] Leunig M, Azegami S, Kamath AF, Ganz R. Femoro-acetabular impingement: Definition, etiology, pathophysiology. In: Nho S, Leunig M, Larson C, Bedi A, Kelly B, editors. Hip Arthroscopy and Hip Joint Preservation Surgery. New York, NY: Springer; 2015

[2] Ganz R, Parvizi J, Beck M, Leunig M, Notzli H, Siebenrock KA. Femoroacetabular impingement: A cause for osteoarthritis of the hip. Clinical Orthopaedics and Related Research. 2003;**417**:112-120

[3] Stulberg SD, Cordell LD, Harris WH, Ramsey PL, MacEwen GD. Unrecognised childhood hip disease: A major cause of idiopathic osteoarthritis of the hip. In: Third Open Scientific Meeting of The Hip Society. St. Louis: CV Mosby Co.; 1975. pp. 212-228

[4] Chaudhry H, Ayeni OR. The etiology of femoroacetabular impingement: What we know and what we don't. Sports Health. 2014;**6**(2):157-161

[5] Mansell NS, Rhon DI, Marchant BG, Slevin JM, Meyer JL. Two-year outcomes after arthroscopic surgery compared to physical therapy for femoracetabular impingement: A protocol for a randomized clinical trial. BMC Musculoskeletal Disorders. 2016;**17**:60

[6] Nakano N, Lisenda L, Jones TL, Loveday DT, Khanduja V. Complications following arthroscopic surgery of the hip: A systematic review of 36 761 cases. Bone & Joint Journal. 2017;**99-B**(12):1577-1583

[7] Malviya A, Raza A, Jameson S, James P, Reed MR, Partington PF. Complications and survival analyses of hip arthroscopies performed in the national health service in England: A review of 6,395 cases. Arthroscopy. 2015;**31**(5):836-842

[8] Harris JD, McCormick FM, Abrams GD, Gupta AK, Ellis TJ, Bach BR Jr, et al. Complications and reoperations during and after hip arthroscopy: A systematic review of 92 studies and more than 6,000 patients. Arthroscopy. 2013;**29**(3):589-595

[9] Griffin DR, Dickenson EJ, O'Donnell J, Agricola R, Awan T, Beck M, et al. The Warwick Agreement on femoroacetabularimpingement syndrome (FAI syndrome): An international consensus statement. British Journal of Sports Medicine. 2016;**50**(19):1169-1176

[10] Raveendran R, Stiller JL, Alvarez C, Renner JB, Schwartz TA, Arden NK, et al. Population-based prevalence of multiple radiographically-defined hip morphologies: The Johnston County osteoarthritis project. Osteoarthritis and Cartilage. 2018;**26**(1):54-61

[11] Hetsroni I, Larson CM, Dela Torre K, Zbeda RM, Magennis E, Kelly BT. Anterior inferior iliac spine deformity as an extra-articular source for hip impingement: A series of 10 patients treated with arthroscopic decompression. Arthroscopy: Journal of Arthroscopic and Related Surgery. 2012;**28**(11):1644-1653

[12] Pan HL, Kawanabe K, Akiyama H, Goto K, Onishi E, Nakamura T. Operative treatment of hip impingement caused by hypertrophy of the anterior inferior iliac spine. The Journal of Bone and Joint Surgery. British Volume. 2008;**90-B**(5):677-679

[13] Aprato A, Giachino M, Masse A. Arthroscopic approach and anatomy of the hip. Muscle, Ligaments and Tendons Journal. 2016;**6**(3):309-316. DOI: 10.11138/mltj/2016.6.3.309

[14] Byrd JW, Pappas JN, Pedley MJ. Hip arthroscopy: An anatomic study of

portal placement and relationship to the extra-articular structures. Arthroscopy. 1995;**11**(4):418-423

[15] Robertson WJ, Kelly BT. The safe zone for hip arthroscopy: A cadaveric assessment of central, peripheral, and lateral compartment portal placement. Arthroscopy. 2008;**24**(9):1019-1026

[16] Larson C, Clohisy J, Beaule P, et al. Complications after hip arthroscopy: A prospective, multicenter study using a validated grading classification. Arthroscopy. 2013;**29**(12 Suppl):e204

[17] Clohisy JC, St John LC, Schutz AL. Surgical treatment of femoroacetabular impingement: A systematic review of the literature. Clinical Orthopaedics and Related Research. 2010;**468**(2):555-564

[18] Cakic J, Patricios J. Femoroacetabular impingement: Prevention or intervention? The sports physician's quandary. British Journal of Sports Medicine. 2014;**48**:1073-1074

[19] Casartelli NC, Maffiuletti NA, Bizzini M, et al. The management of symptomatic femoroacetabular impingement: What is the rationale for non-surgical treatment? British Journal of Sports Medicine. 2016;**50**:511-512

[20] Papavasiliou AV, Bardakos NV. Complications of arthroscopic surgery of the hip. Bone & Joint Research. 2012;**1**:131-144

Chapter 3

Arthroscopic and Endoscopic Management of the Internal Snapping Hip Syndrome

Adinun Apivatgaroon

Abstract

Internal snapping hip syndrome or coxa saltans interna results from the iliopsoas tendon snapping over the superior pubic ramus, iliopectineal eminence, anterior hip joint, femoral head or the lesser trochanter. This condition occurs in either the native hip or a prosthetic hip joint. Conservative management is the mainstay treatment, but iliopsoas release continues to be the definitive treatment in patients with failed conservative measures. The arthroscopic iliopsoas release from the central or peripheral compartment is useful in the management of internal snapping syndrome and may have less hip flexion strength deficits postoperatively as compared to the releasing from the lesser trochanteric level. Endoscopic iliopsoas release at the lesser trochanter level is the preferred operative treatment option for internal snapping patients who have undergone a total hip replacement.

Keywords: internal snapping hip syndrome, iliopsoas impingement, coxa saltans interna, iliopsoas release

1. Introduction

Snapping hip syndrome or coxa saltans is an abnormal hip condition that includes a painful popping sensation and sound with movement around the hip joint. In the general population, snapping hip can be found in about 5–10% and for most are asymptomatic. Snapping hip syndrome can be divided as intra-articular and extra-articular snapping as seen in **Table 1**.

Internal snapping hip syndrome is snapping hip caused by the iliopsoas tendon migrating over the superior pubic ramus, iliopectineal eminence, anterior hip joint, femoral head or the lesser trochanter. Multiple or bifid iliopsoas tendons can also be found during transcapsular iliopsoas release in about 17.85% of cases [1].

Signs and symptoms include pain or a popping sensation in the area near the anterior groin. The clicking or popping sensation can be reproduced by allowing the patient to perform active hip extension and/or external rotation in a flexion position of the hip (**Figure 1**). Some patients present with a positive C-sign at the painful area. The patients may have focal tenderness over the iliopsoas (anterior groin) and a positive impingement test (Flexion-Adduction-Internal Rotation test, FADIR test) either with or without concomitant femoroacetabular impingement syndrome.

The resisted straight leg raise (RSLR) test is performed by the patient flexing the hip actively at approximately 30° in full knee extension. The examiner places a hand just above the patient's knee to resist hip flexion in that position (**Figure 2**).

Intra-articular snapping	Extra-articular snapping
Soft tissue • Labral tears • Ligamentum teres rupture, impingement	Anterior or internal • Iliopsoas snapping (internal snapping hip) Lateral or external • Iliotibial band snapping (external snapping hip)
Bone and cartilage • Chondral damage • Loose bodies • Chondromatosis • Femoroacetabular impingement (FAI)	

Table 1.
Approach of the snapping hip syndrome that can be divided as intra-articular and extra-articular causes.

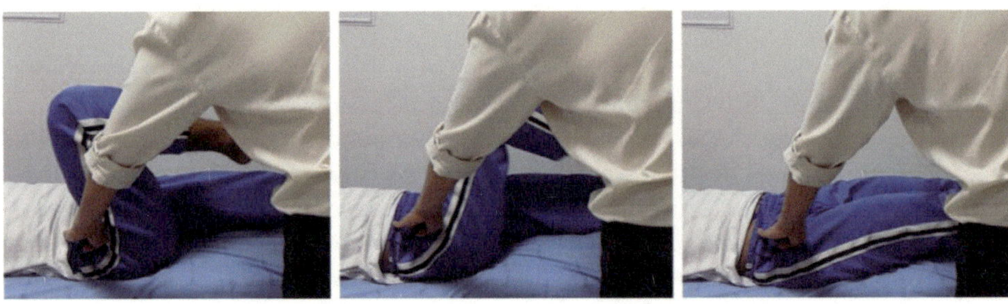

Figure 1.
The internal snapping test is performed by letting the patient performs active hip extension and/or external rotation from the starting flexion position of the examined hip. Positive result when the clicking or popping sensation can be reproduced.

A positive result is when there is pain at the anterior groin or weakness in the hip flexion that represents iliopsoas problems or intra-articular pathologies [2].

The investigations include plain radiographs of the pelvis/hip that might be helpful in ruling out other causes of hip pain or detecting associated pathologies that can affect the hip joint. MRI of the affected hip could aid in ruling out others causes of hip pain or detect associated pathologies, particularly, an anterior labral lesion. Some studies showed the correlation of a 3 O'clock positioned labral tear/injury with iliopsoas impingement by the friction of the iliopsoas tendon to the predominately, anterior portion of the labrum caused tear [3, 4]. Dynamic ultrasonography is useful to detect snapping of the iliopsoas during actual hip motion and can be conjugate with an ultrasound-guided bursal injection. In iliopsoas impingement, the pain could be improved after an iliopsoas bursal injection rather than an intra-articular injection of anesthetic agents [4].

Nowadays, total hip replacements (THR) are increasing in numbers and indications [5]. An iliopsoas impingement can be a complication of this procedure from impingement of the iliopsoas tendon with the acetabular component [6, 7] (**Figure 3**). This is noticeable in the large size of the acetabular components or in patients with dysplastic morphology of the native hip associated with under coverage of the anterior/superior acetabular rim.

Conservative management of internal snapping hip syndrome includes rest, activity modification, anti-inflammatory medications, injections of a local anesthetic combined with a corticosteroid into the involved bursa or around the tendon sheath and the stretching of the iliopsoas (**Figure 4**).

The surgical treatment consists of iliopsoas release via an open, arthroscopic or endoscopic approach with or without intra-articular procedures. In the total hip

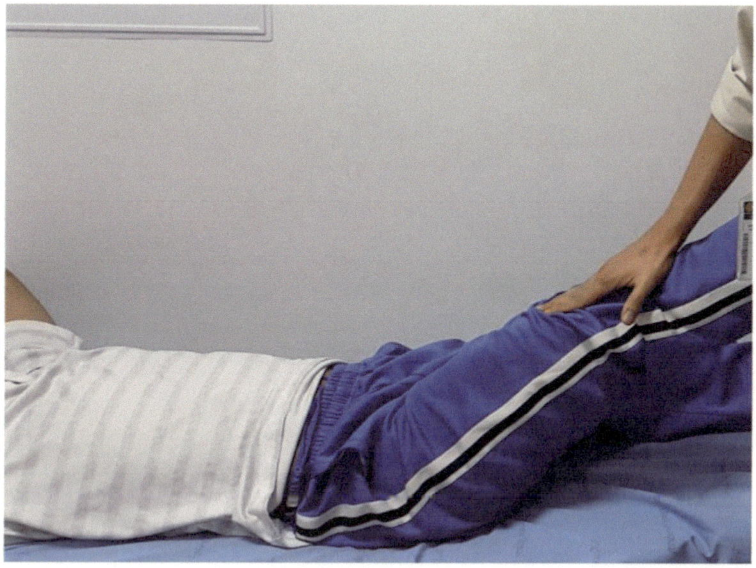

Figure 2.
The resisted straight leg raise (RSLR) test is performed by allowing the patient flex to the hip actively to approximately 30° in a full knee extension, the examiner places a hand just above the patient's knee to resist hip flexion in that position. Positive result when pain or weakness represents iliopsoas pathology or intra-articular causes.

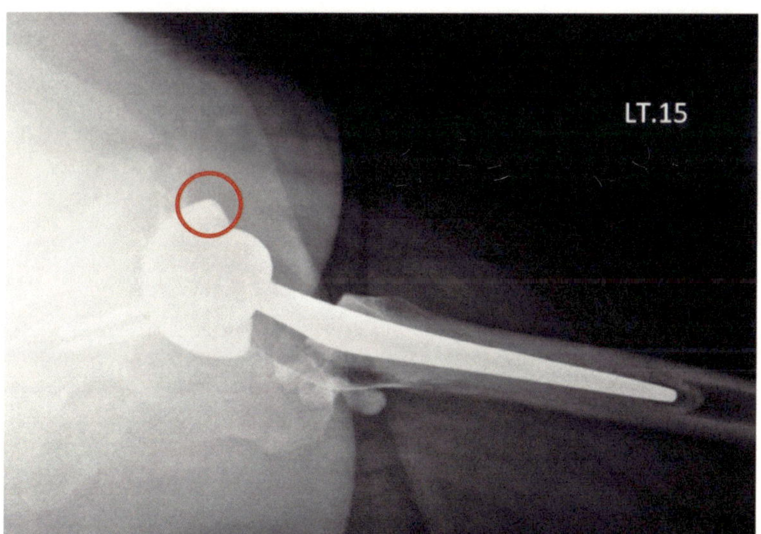

Figure 3.
A lateral cross table radiograph of the left hip following total hip arthroplasty demonstrates the anterior overhang of the acetabular component (red circle) at about 5 mm, leading to iliopsoas impingement.

replacement patient with obvious acetabular component malposition or prominence, acetabular cup revision maybe necessary [6]. For the arthroscopic/endoscopic iliopsoas release techniques, these can be performed using: 1. the transcapsular release (proximal arthroscopic release) via the central or peripheral compartment and 2. releasing at the lesser trochanteric level (distal endoscopic release) (**Figure 5**).

In this chapter, two common iliopsoas release procedures will be presented. The contents of indications, patients positioning, arthroscopic/endoscopic portals and

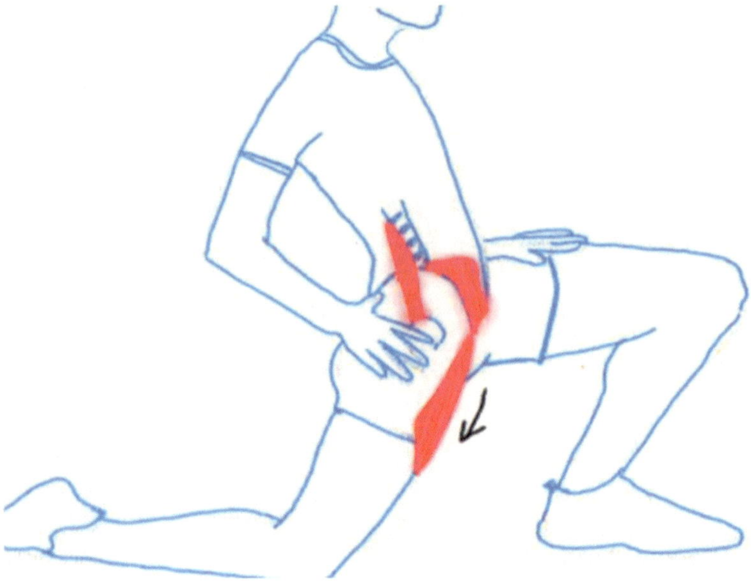

Figure 4.
Demonstrate the stretching method of the right iliopsoas muscle/tendon. The affected hip is extended during controlled trunk balancing.

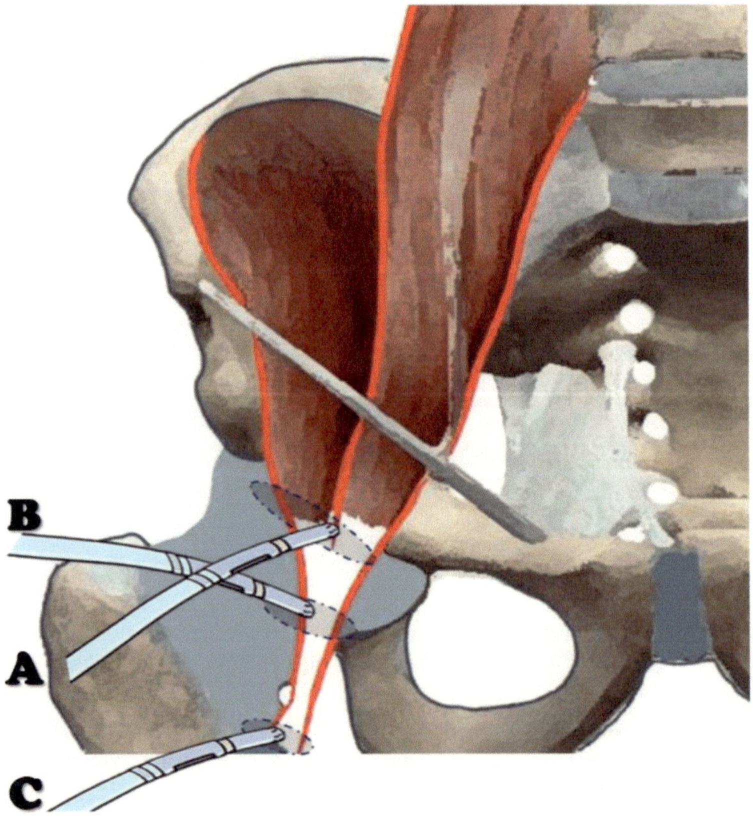

Figure 5.
Demonstration of the iliopsoas release techniques: (A) proximal arthroscopic transcapsular release via a central compartment approach; (B) proximal arthroscopic transcapsular release via a peripheral compartment approach; and (c) distal endoscopic release at the lesser trochanteric level.

the details of procedures are described. The evidence-based reviews of the procedures will also be presented.

2. Arthroscopic transcapsular release (proximal arthroscopic release)

2.1 Indications

- Internal snapping hip syndrome with failed conservative treatments for more than 4–6 months.
- Conjugate with the arthroscopic procedure of the hip (such as anterior labral repair).

2.2 Patient position

The iliopsoas release could be performed using the supine or lateral decubitus position. The author's preferred patient position is supine on a traction radiolucent table (Maquet, Rastatt, Germany). Both legs and feet are well padded and wrapped with soft cotton and hung on the footplate. A large, well-padded perineal post is used to prevent complications from pudendal nerve compression. The C-arm is placed at the non-operative side and positioned horizontally to check the anteroposterior view of the affected hip. Traction is performed to check the possibility of central compartment assess and intra-articular arthroscopic work.

2.3 Surgical technique

The peripheral compartment approach is introduced in hip flexion of 20–30° using a proximal anterolateral portal (PAL). Peripheral compartment examination and synovectomy are performed using an anterior working portal (**Figure 6**). Following the peripheral compartment work that includes synovectomy and cam resection, the central compartment is assessed under traction of the hip in a full extension position. Intra-articular examination and surgical procedures are completely performed. These include; debridement, acetabuloplasty, and labral surgery.

The arthroscopic iliopsoas tenotomy can performed by two methods: (1) central compartment approach under traction and (2) peripheral compartment approach with hip flexion of 20–30°.

In a central compartment approach. After performing the intra-articular procedures, the arthroscope is retracted to the peripheral compartment to assess under traction the anterior hip capsule at approximately the 3 O'clock position of the anterior labrum. This step uses the anterolateral viewing portal and the anterior portal for the procedure. Inflammation of the anterior labrum may represent evidence of iliopsoas impingement. The iliopsoas tendon is located near the anteromedial aspect of the anterior hip capsule. The anterior capsule at this area is thin and some patients have an anterior capsular hole directly connected to the iliopsoas tendon [8]. A capsulotomy of approximately 1–2 cm is performed to the 3 O'clock position of the right hip. After capsulotomy, the synovial tissue around the iliopsoas tendon is identified and resected using an arthroscopic shaver or electrocautery. The iliopsoas tendon is identified and released until the iliacus muscle can be observed beneath the released portion of the tendon. Keeping this portion of the iliacus muscle may decrease of the risk of hip flexion weakness, postoperatively (**Figure 7**).

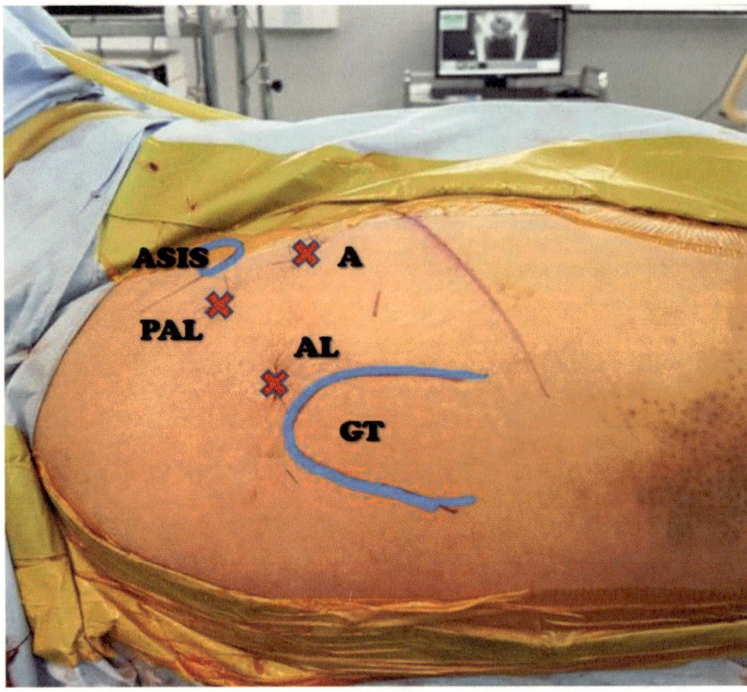

Figure 6.
The portals used in peripheral compartment approach of the right hip. Proximal anterolateral portal (PAL) is the start and viewing portal. Anterior (A) and anterolateral (AL) portals are shown. GT, greater trochanter; ASIS, anterior superior iliac spine.

In the peripheral compartment approach, following the intra-articular work, the traction is released to reduce the hip joint. The arthroscope is inserted via the same AL viewing portal or re-inserted from the PAL portal in the hip at 20–30° in a flexion position. Then, the zona orbicularis, medial synovial fold, and the anterior labrum are identified. The medial synovial fold is the landmark for the most inferomedial head–neck area, also known as, the 6 O'clock position. The 1–2 cm capsulotomy is performed at the capsular space between the anterior labrum and the zona orbicularis close to the proximal attachment of the medial synovial fold. After capsulotomy, the synovial tissue around the iliopsoas tendon is resected as previously described and the iliopsoas tendon is released while preserving the iliacus muscle.

It is not necessary to perform the capsular closure if the capsulotomy is less than 1–2 cm. With complete tenotomy of the iliopsoas, either in the central or peripheral approach, the portals are sutured simple and the wounds are closed in standard fashion.

2.4 Post-operative rehabilitation

Active hip range of motion is allowed immediately post operatively. The hip flexion strength may decrease in the first 6 to 8 weeks and usually restores after 8 weeks. Active hip flexor strengthening exercises are allowed after 6 weeks postoperatively.

Weight bearing is dependent on the intra-articular conditions. The patients apply partial weight bearing for 6 weeks if the cartilage or the labral lesions were repaired/fixated, or if osteochondroplasty of the cam lesion is done. In the isolated iliopsoas release patients, there is no need to protect weight bearing after post operatively. Return to sport activities are allowed after 3 months.

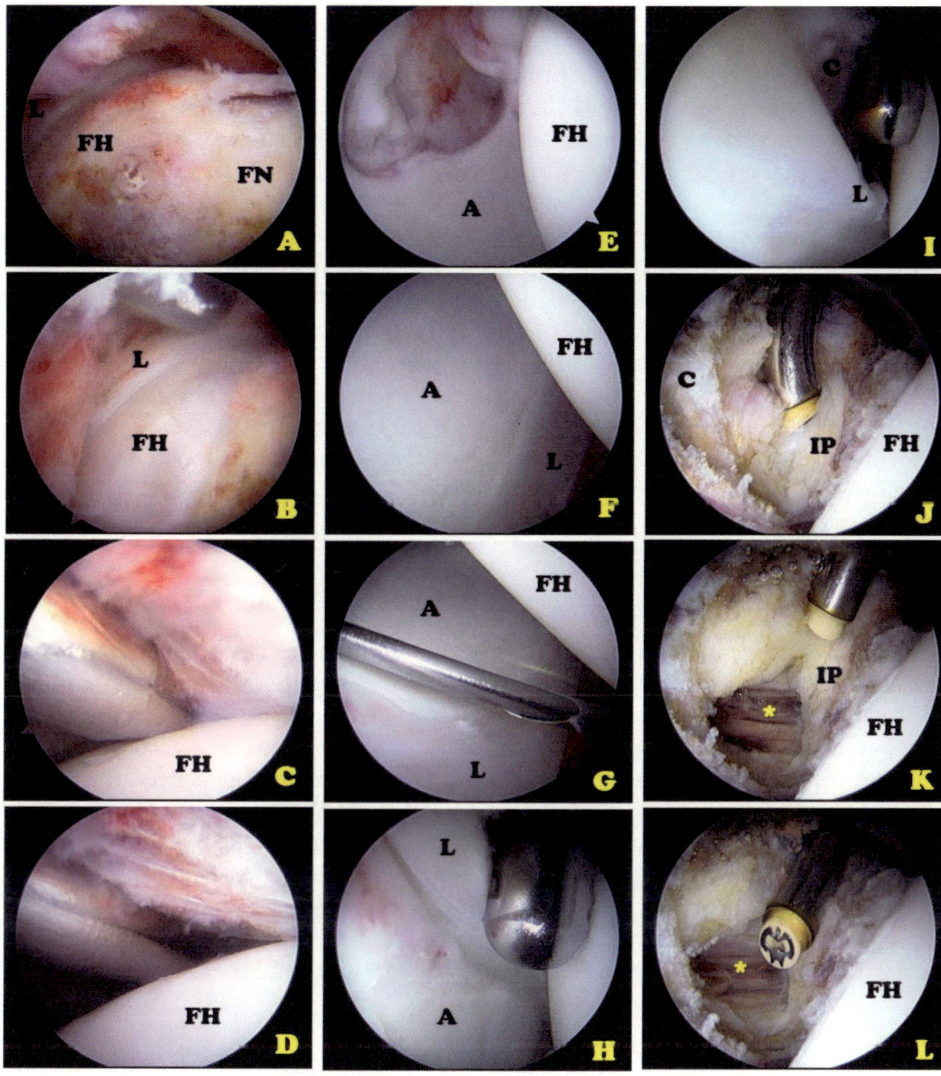

Figure 7.
Arthroscopic view of the central compartment transcapsular iliopsoas tenotomy of the right hip. (A and B) Peripheral compartment first approach using the proximal anterolateral (PAL) viewing portal and anterior working portal. (C and D) Approach to the central compartment by direct visualization and inserting the switching stick through the anterior portal. (E and F) Examination in the central compartment. (G) Create the anterolateral (AL) portal under direct visualization using anterior viewing portal. (H and I) Switch the scope to the AL viewing portal and working from the anterior portal. (J to L) After a small anterior capsulotomy to about the 3 O'clock position, the iliopsoas tendon (IP) is cut using electrocautery. The iliacus muscle (*) is preserved. [L-labrum, FH-femoral head, FN-femoral neck, A-acetabulum, C-capsule].

3. Endoscopic iliopsoas release at the lesser trochanteric level (distal endoscopic release)

3.1 Indications

- Painful iliopsoas impingement following a total hip replacement, no obvious malposition of the acetabular cup and the anterior overhang is <8 mm.
- Failed conservative more than 4–6 months with positive iliopsoas injection test.
- No evidence of prosthesis loosening or infection.

3.2 Patient position

Preoperative physical examination, blood analysis for white blood cell count, erythrocyte sedimentation rate (ESR) and C-reactive protein (CRP), hip X-rays, and CT assessment are needed to evaluate possible other causes of hip/groin pain in total hip replacement patients. Infection and prosthesis loosening need to be ruled out.

The author's preferred patient position is supine on a radiolucent traction table (Maquet, Rastatt, Germany) similar for the patient with an arthroscopic proximal release. Both legs and feet are well padded, wrapped with soft cotton and hung to the footplate. A large, well-padded perineal post is used to prevent complications from pudendal nerve compression. The C-arm is placed at the non-operative side and positioned horizontally to check the anteroposterior view of the affected hip. Traction of the prosthetic component is not a requirement and the release is performed at the lesser trochanter level. The affected leg is placed in an externally rotated position of the hip in full knee extension. This moves the lesser trochanter further anteriorly (**Figure 8**).

3.3 Surgical technique

The endoscopic portals are marked as seen in **Figure 9**. The anterolateral portal (1–2 cm anterior to level of tip of greater trochanter) and distal anterolateral portal (5–7 cm distal to anterolateral portal) are identified. The direction of the instrument and arthroscope can be aligned under fluoroscopic control toward the tip of the lesser trochanter (**Figure 10**). The needle and guidewire are inserted through the anterolateral portal with the designed trajectory toward the lesser trochanter. A 4.5-mm cannulated switching-stick (Smith and Nephew, MA, USA) is inserted then changed to a 5.0-mm cannula and an obturator. Blunt dissection using the cannula is performed above the lesser trochanter in a superior-inferior direction to create more working space anteriorly under fluoroscopic guidance. A 70° arthroscope is inserted via this anterolateral portal and the distal anterolateral portal is created as a second

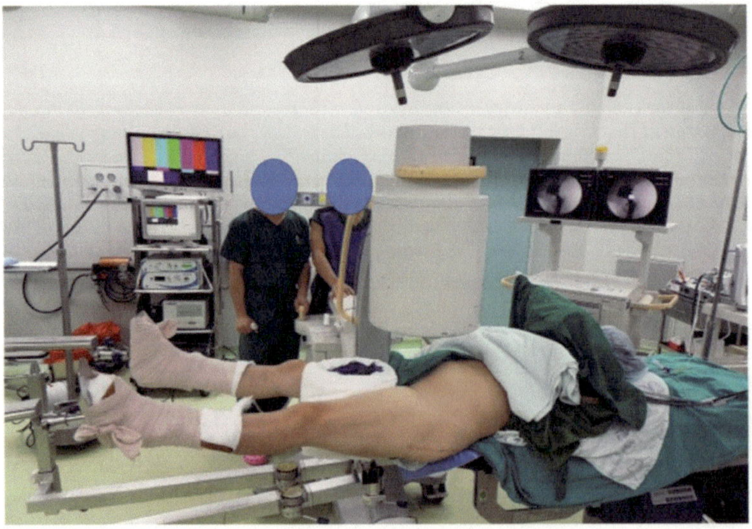

Figure 8.
Patient positioned for the endoscopic iliopsoas release of the left hip. Supine on the radiolucent traction table. The surgical hip is in external rotation, fully stretched in full knee extension that brings the lessor trochanter further anteriorly.

DOI: http://dx.doi.org/10.5772/intechopen.91919

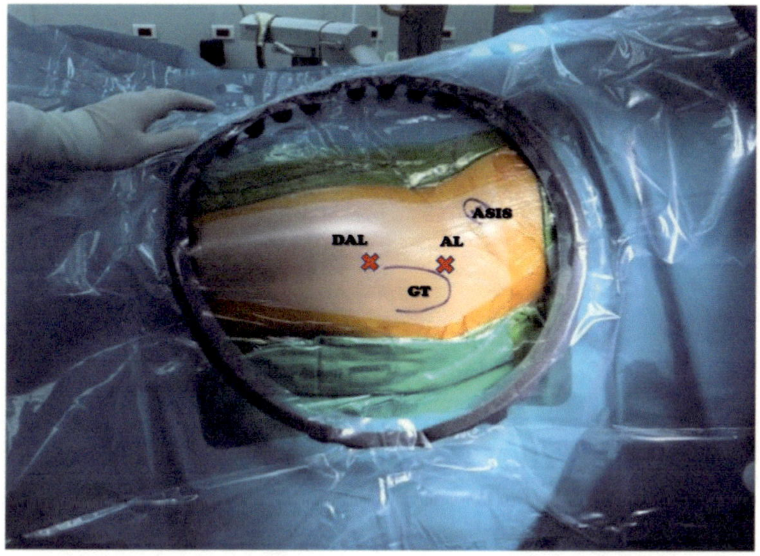

Figure 9.
Endoscopic portals of the left hip in supine position without traction. Left hand is patient's up and right is the legs. AL, anterolateral portal; DAL, distal anterolateral portal; ASIS, anterior superior iliac spine; GT, greater trochanter.

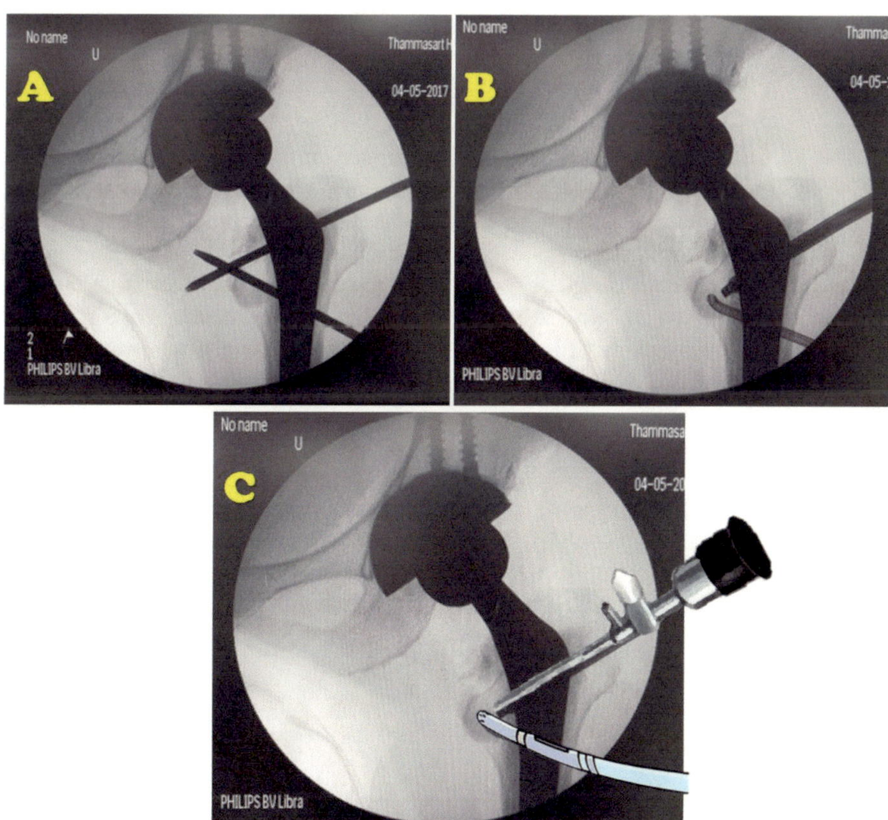

Figure 10.
Demonstration of the direction of the instrument and endoscope under fluoroscopic control in a left, prosthetic hip: (A) both instruments aimed toward tip of the lessor trochanter in the convergence direction. (B) and (C) the endoscope is inserted from the AL portal and the radiofrequency abrasion is inserted from the DAL portal.

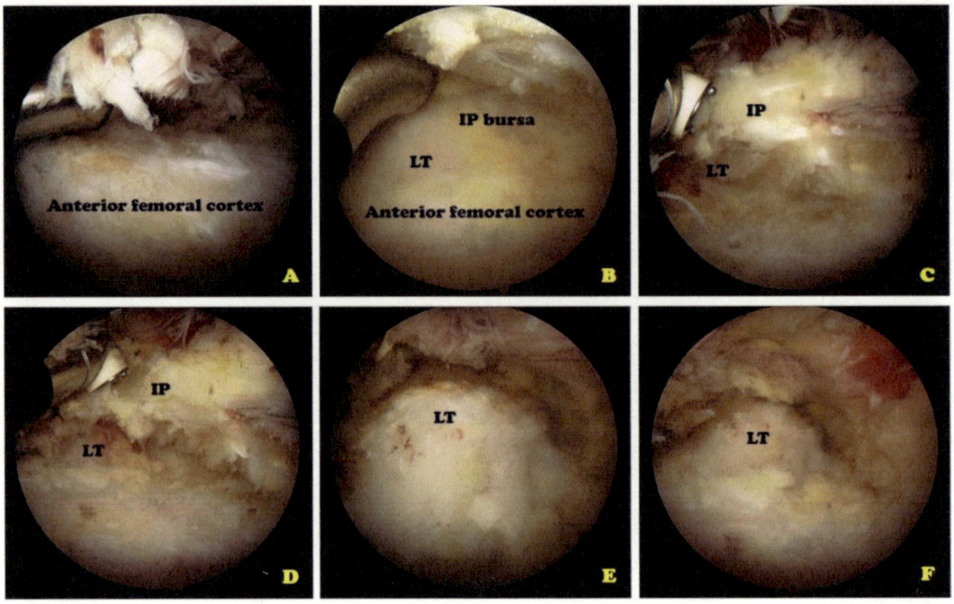

Figure 11.
Endoscopic view from the anterolateral portal of the left hip; right is the proximal aspect and left is the distal aspect of the proximal femur: (A) and (B) identification of the anterior femoral cortex, iliopsoas bursa (IP bursa) and lessor trochanter (LT) using the distal anterolateral working portal; (C) identification of the iliopsoas tendon (IP) which attaches to the lessor trochanter; (D) peeled-off iliopsoas tendon from the lessor trochanter using radiofrequency; and (E) and (F) lessor trochanter and the surrounding tissue after the iliopsoas tendon release.

portal using a needle and guidewire under fluoroscopy. The 4.5-mm, cannulated switching stick is inserted through the guidewire under endoscopic control. The iliopsoas tendon is identified at the lesser trochanteric insertion then, the radiofrequency or an arthroscopic shaver is used via the distal anterolateral portal to remove the iliopsoas bursa surrounding the tendon and to obtain adequate visualization of the tendon. The iliopsoas tendon is 'peeled' from the lesser trochanter using radiofrequency under direct vision (**Figure 11**). After completion of the tenotomy, the portals are simply sutured, and the wounds are closed in standard fashion.

3.4 Postoperative rehabilitation

Active hip range of motion exercises are allowed immediately following surgery. Hip flexion strength may decrease in the first 6–8 weeks and usually returns to baseline after 8 weeks. Active hip flexor strengthening exercises are allowed after 6 weeks postoperative. The patients progress to full weight bearing as soon as possible, postoperatively. Return to normal activities is allowed 6–8 weeks after surgery.

4. Discussion

An iliopsoas tenotomy has shown good to excellent postoperative outcomes in indicated patients with iliopsoas snapping/impingement. The systematic reviews of 11 eligible studies (248 patients), level IV studies revealed 'the resolution of snapping' as seen in 100% of patients who underwent an arthroscopic release and 77% of those who underwent open procedures. The complication rates were higher in patients undergoing an open procedure (21%) compared with an arthroscopic procedure (2.3%). The analysis of the open procedure; either open transection of the iliopsoas tendon at the level of the lesser trochanter (14 patients) or open tendon lengthening of the iliopsoas tendon (105 patients) has shown 27 of 119 patients with recurrence of snapping and 4 of 119 experienced snapping with pain, 6 patients needed a second surgical intervention. There was an increased prevalence of recurrent snapping with open transection of the iliopsoas tendon as compared to patients with iliopsoas tendon lengthening (43% vs. 20%). The complications of the open procedure are postoperative pain (11–36%) and the hip flexion weakness (8–14%). In the arthroscopic group with transection at the lesser trochanter and transcapsular release, 3 of 37 (8%) patients of the group with transection at lesser trochanter reported complications including 2 cases of ischial bursitis and 1 case of greater trochanteric bursitis. No reported complications from the transcapsular release group. No hip flexion weakness was reported in the arthroscopic groups. None of the arthroscopically treated patients required a second surgical intervention [9].

A study of 25 patients with 2-year follow up following transcapsular release with intra-articular procedures in the internal snapping hip with combined pathologies revealed 88% of patients with good to excellent results without serious complications [10]. A comparative case-series with 20 patients, including 6 patients with a release at the lesser trochanter level vs. 14 central compartment release patients revealed the same favorable results based-on WOMAC scores. Just 1 of 14 patient with central compartment release had a recurrence of snapping that required surgical intervention. No complications were reported in both groups [11].

The iliopsoas release/tenotomy is the treatment option for iliopsoas tendinopathy or impingement following a total hip replacement. A systematic review of level IV studies in 18 studies (11 case series, 6 case reports and 1 prospective cohort) of 171 patients who underwent hip arthroscopy after an arthroplasty revealed the pathology, including 35.8% of iliopsoas tendinopathy, 24.6% of symptomatic hips with no clear diagnosis, 6.4% of periprosthetic infection, and 3.5% of intra-articular loose bodies. Almost all patients who underwent hip arthroscopy experienced positive outcomes from the procedure [12]. A systematic review of 11 studies, 280 hips treated for iliopsoas impingement, following a total hip replacement, showed improved outcome scores in all three treatment groups including: 1. conservative treatment group (54 patients using local injections and physical therapy), 2. Iliopsoas tenotomy group (133 patients using either arthroscopic, endoscopic or an open approach), and 3. Revision arthroplasty (93 patients by exchange of the acetabular component). The tenotomy group reported 5 (3.76%) complications that included 1 patient with a 13-mm acetabular prominence with continuing groin pain and subsequently needed component revision, 1 patient with a heterotrophic ossification, 1 anterior dislocation, 1 compressive hematoma affecting the peroneal nerve, and 1 periprosthetic ossification. The revision arthroplasty group reported 18 (19.4%) complications including 5 developing trochanteric bursitis, 4 with recurrent groin pain, 2 revision surgeries, 2 dislocations, 1 DVT, 1 deep infection, 1 trochanteric nonunion, 1 superficial wound infection, and 1 disarticulation [13].

A retrospective review of 49 patients [6] who had been treated for iliopsoas impingement after a primary total hip arthroplasty with 4 years of mean follow-up show 50% (10 patients) in the nonoperative group had groin pain resolution as compared to 76% (22 patients) in the operative group ($p = 0.06$). The patients with <8 mm of component prominent tenotomy stated 100% resolution of groin pain (5 patients) but patients with ≥8 mm of prominent tenotomy led to groin pain resolution at only 33% (3 patients). Acetabular revision in patients with ≥8 mm of prominence had groin pain resolution in 92% (12 of 13 patients) ($p = 0.07$). Thus, it is suggested that use of tenotomy in patients with <8 mm of component prominence and acetabular revision in patients with ≥8 mm of prominence is indicated.

5. Conclusion

Iliopsoas snapping is one of the causes of hip pain in either, native or prosthetic hips. The mainstay treatment is conservative management, especially, in iliopsoas stretching. The iliopsoas release is the definite treatment in failed conservative patients. Either arthroscopic iliopsoas release from the central/peripheral compartment or, endoscopic iliopsoas release at the lesser trochanter level have shown good to excellent results in the postoperative outcomes. Acetabular revision may be considered in patients with ≥8 mm of prominence with persistent groin pain following a total hip replacement.

Acknowledgements

The author thanks the Orthopedics Department, Faculty of Medicine, Thammasat University and Thammasat University Hospital for the kind support. No funding was obtained regarding this manuscript.

Conflict of interest

The authors declare no conflict of interest.

Appendices and nomenclature

internal snapping hip syndrome
coxa saltans interna
iliopectineal eminence
arthroscopic iliopsoas release
endoscopic iliopsoas release
total hip replacement

Author details

Adinun Apivatgaroon
Orthopaedics Department, Thammasat University, Thailand

*Address all correspondence to: adino_ball@yahoo.com

References

[1] Ilizaliturri VM Jr, Suarez-Ahedo C, Acuña M. Internal snapping hip syndrome: Incidence of multiple-tendon existence and outcome after endoscopic transcapsular release. Arthroscopy. 2015;**31**(10):1991-1995

[2] Troelsen A, Mechlenburg I, Gelineck J, Bolvig L, Jacobsen S, Søballe K. What is the role of clinical tests and ultrasound in acetabular labral tear diagnostics? Acta Orthopaedica. 2009;**80**(3):314-318

[3] Blankenbaker DG, Tuite MJ, Keene JS, del Rio AM. Labral injuries due to iliopsoas impingement: Can they be diagnosed on MR arthrography? American Journal of Roentgenology. 2012;**199**(4):894-900

[4] Domb BG, Shindle MK, McArthur B, Voos JE, Magennis EM, Kelly BT. Iliopsoas impingement: A newly identified cause of labral pathology in the hip. HSS Journal. 2011;7(2):145-150

[5] Singh JA, Yu S, Chen L, Cleveland JD. Rates of total joint replacement in the United States: Future projections to 2020-2040 using the National Inpatient Sample. The Journal of Rheumatology. 2019;**46**(9):1134-1140

[6] Chalmers BP, Sculco PK, Sierra RJ, Trousdale RT, Berry DJ. Iliopsoas impingement after primary total hip arthroplasty: Operative and nonoperative treatment outcomes. The Journal of Bone and Joint Surgery. American Volume. 2017;**99**(7):557-564

[7] Guicherd W, Bonin N, Gicquel T, Gedouin JE, Flecher X, Wettstein M, et al. Endoscopic or arthroscopic iliopsoas tenotomy for iliopsoas impingement following total hip replacement. A prospective multicenter 64-case series. Orthopaedics & Traumatology, Surgery & Research. 2017;**103**(8S):S207-S214

[8] Wettstein M, Jung J, Dienst M. Arthroscopic psoas tenotomy. Arthroscopy. 2006;**22**(8):907.e1-4

[9] Khan M, Philippon MJ, et al. Surgical management of internal snapping hip syndrome: A systematic review evaluating open and arthroscopic approaches. Arthroscopy. 2013;**29**(5):942-948

[10] Hwang DS, Hwang JM, Kim PS, Rhee SM, Park SH, Kang SY, et al. Arthroscopic treatment of symptomatic internal snapping hip with combined pathologies. Clinics in Orthopedic Surgery. 2015;**7**(2):158-163

[11] Ilizaliturri VM Jr, Buganza-Tepole M, Olivos-Meza A, Acuna M, Acosta-Rodriguez E. Central compartment release versus lesser trochanter release of the iliopsoas tendon for the treatment of internal snapping hip: A comparative study. Arthroscopy. 2014;**30**(7):790-795

[12] Heaven S, de Sa D, Simunovic N, Williams DS, Naudie D, Ayeni OR. Hip arthroscopy in the setting of hip arthroplasty. Knee Surgery, Sports Traumatology, Arthroscopy. 2016;**24**(1):287-294

[13] Shapira J, Chen SL, Wojnowski NM, Lall AC, Rosinsky PJ, Maldonado DR, et al. Outcomes of nonoperative management, iliopsoas tenotomy, and revision arthroplasty for Iliopsoas impingement after total hip arthroplasty: A systematic review. The Journal of Arthroplasty. 2019;**34**(9):2184-2191

Chapter 4

The Practice of Computer-Assisted Planning and Navigation for Hip Arthroscopy

Naomi Kobayashi, Shota Higashihira and Yutaka Inaba

Abstract

Despite significant developments in hip arthroscopic surgery in recent years, precise preoperative planning and accurate performance remain challenging. Preoperative planning is particularly important in cases of osteochondroplasty for cam-type femoroacetabular impingement (FAI), and can be aided by several computer-assisted tools, including three-dimensional imaging analysis or kinematic analysis. Initially, the exact point of the bony impingement is identified using simulation analysis; then, virtual osteochondroplasty is performed. Improvements in the range of motion can then be evaluated using computer simulation again. In this way, the required area and depth of bone resection can be assessed preoperatively. In addition, computed tomography-based navigation assistance can be used to complete the osteochondroplasty in accordance with the preoperative planning. After surgery, postoperative evaluation provides valuable feedback to improve future planning and procedures. In this chapter, we describe the practice of computer-assisted planning and navigation for hip arthroscopy.

Keywords: hip arthroscopy, femoroacetabular impingement, computer-assisted surgery, navigation

1. Introduction

In the last decade, hip arthroscopic surgery has become widely recognized as an effective option for the treatment of femoroacetabular impingement (FAI). In order to achieve optimal clinical results, it is essential to correct the bony impingement, and therefore, precise osteochondroplasty is one of the most important factors. However, it is not possible to predict the impingement point in each case based only on radiographic images [1]; and computer simulation modeling is important to provide three-dimensional identification. This is the starting point of computer-assisted hip arthroscopy; thereafter, preoperative planning is conducted by virtual osteochondroplasty in a computer model, before transferring to a navigation system. Therefore, the computer-assisted tool not only provides surgical assistance, but also supports the preoperative planning. The real value of the computer navigation system lies in the ability to undertake precise preoperative planning, and it is difficult to achieve precise and reliable surgical results without computer navigation. After surgery, the area of impingement can be re-evaluated using postoperative computed tomography (CT) data. Furthermore, it is possible to validate the

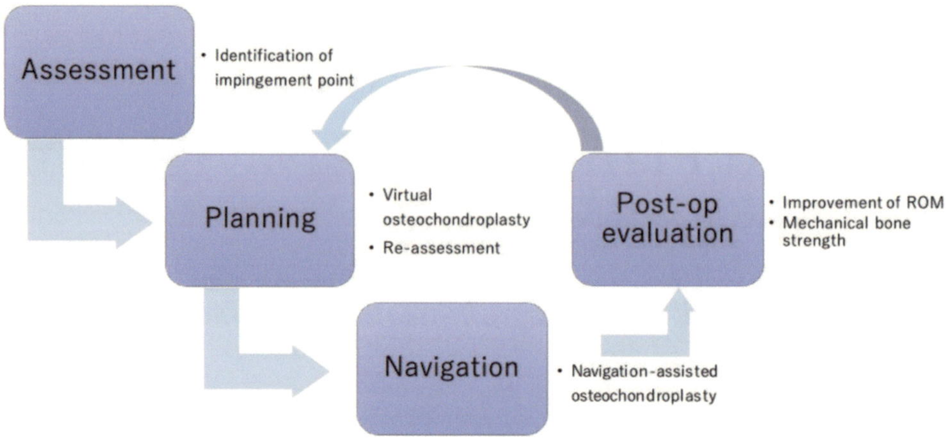

Figure 1.
Flow of computer-assisted hip arthroscopy for FAI.

mechanical bone strength after osteochondroplasty using finite element analysis. These postoperative evaluations provide important feedback for future cases, as illustrated in **Figure 1**.

2. Identification of impingement points

The distribution of impingement points in cam lesions is dependent on the morphology in each femoral head-neck junction, as well as acetabular morphology, such as dysplasia [2]. Bone-to-bone impingement occurs during the dynamic phase of hip motion, such as flexion and internal rotation. Therefore, it is not possible to identify the impingement point by radiograph only. Computer modeling based on CT data allows the identification of the exact impingement point in each lower limb position. As a representative position for anterior impingement, maximum internal rotation at a 90° flexion is preferred for impingement simulation (**Figure 2**). The ZedHip (Lexi, Tokyo) system is used for the computer simulation analysis. It is important to note that the impingement point is dependent on the hip position setting, i.e., flexion angle or additional adduction of the hip. The position setting is

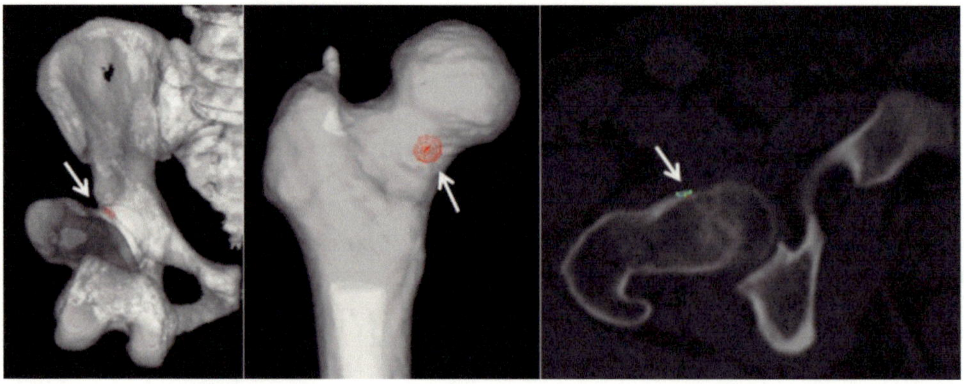

Figure 2.
Identification of the impingement point by computer simulation. Impingement simulation with 90° flexion and maximum internal rotation is conducted. The impingement point is identified in the three-dimensional femur model and axial image (arrow).

variable, and it is difficult to define the optimal setting, which is one of the limitations of this approach, as discussed later in this chapter.

In a previous study by Oishi et al. [3], impingement simulation was applied and compared with the abnormal uptake point by positron emission tomography. This study showed that impingement may occur more frequently at <90° flexion in patients with FAI syndrome with cam morphology. In addition, the range of hip motion in daily life is activity-dependent. Therefore, further evaluation is required to establish the appropriate hip position setting for impingement simulation representing the variety of hip positions during different activities associated with daily life.

3. Virtual osteochondroplasty and assessment of improved range of motion

The next step in the preoperative planning process is computerized "virtual osteochondroplasty" (**Figure 3**). The bony region is deleted in the editing mode of the ZedHip software with the central focus on the impingement point. It is important to delete the bony region smoothly, rather than creating a notch, as it is with the actual osteochondroplasty. Flexion angle at 70 or 45° should be added as a simulation condition. It should be noted that virtual osteochondroplasty should be performed using the same assumptions as actual surgery, i.e., excessive osteochondroplasty should be avoided to maintain bone strength. A previous study using an animal model of mechanical testing and finite element analysis revealed that up to 36% of the femoral neck diameter could be safely resected during simulated osteochondroplasty [4]. By contrast, residual cam deformity is one of the most important risk factors for revision surgery [5]. It is, therefore, important to pay close attention to the trade-off between bone strength and the risk of residual deformity.

After deleting the impinging bony region during virtual osteochondroplasty, a bone model is reconstructed. Using this model, the range of motion can be re-evaluated and compared with the situation prior to virtual osteochondroplasty. It is difficult to judge the improvement in maximum internal rotation angle; however, we suggest that the threshold is set at 10°. Therefore, virtual osteochondroplasty should be performed until an improvement of more than 10° is confirmed. Kubota et al. evaluated the improvement of range of motion after virtual osteochondroplasty, comparing FAI and borderline dysplasia cases [6]. **Figure 4** shows the difference in improvement between cam-type FAI and borderline dysplasia with or without

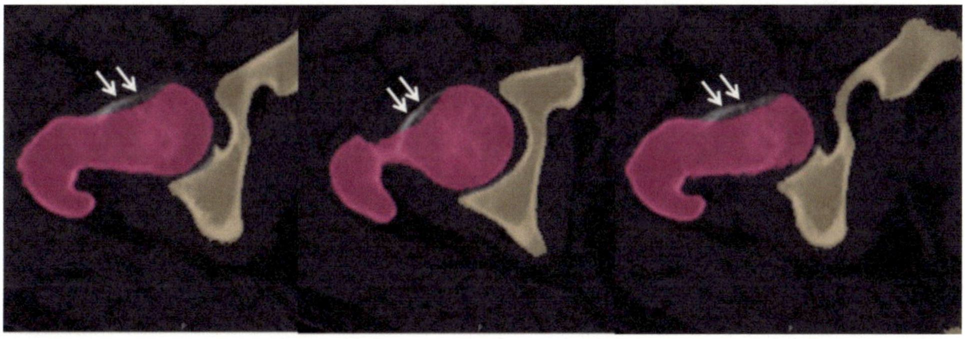

Figure 3.
Virtual osteochondroplasty in preoperative planning. With the central focus on the impingement point, osteochondroplasty is performed in the computer simulation model. The purple colored area shows the post-resected bone region; bone resection must be conducted smoothly to avoid creating a notch (arrows).

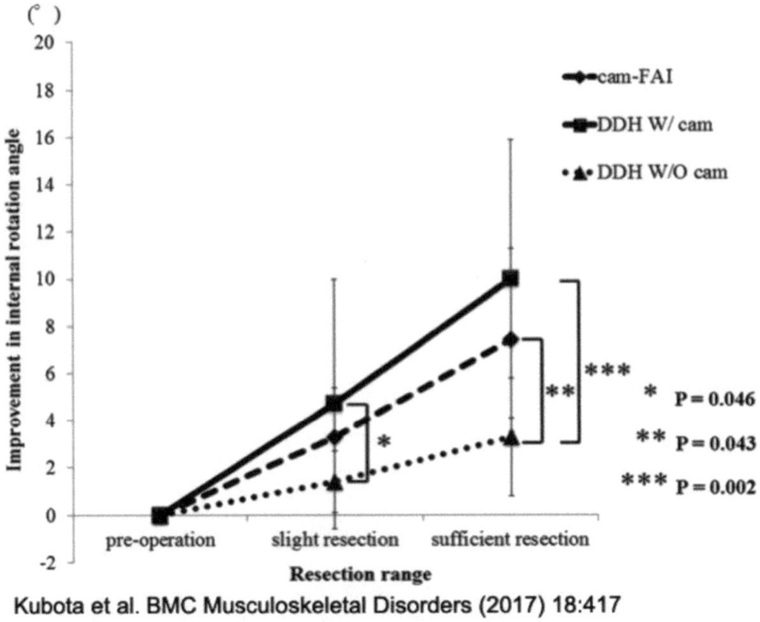

Figure 4.
Improvement in the internal rotation angle after each type of resection. The mean improvement in the internal rotation angle in the DDH with cam group after slight resection was significantly greater than that in the DDH without cam group (P = 0.046), as was that after sufficient resection (P = 0.002). The improvement in the cam-FAI group was significantly greater than that in the DDH without cam group (P = 0.043). DDH: developmental dysplasia of the hip.

cam morphology [6], demonstrating that the improvement in the range of motion is dependent on the extent of bone resection. An interesting clinical implication in this study is that borderline dysplasia with cam morphology showed the most significant improvement by virtual osteochondroplasty. Therefore, even in cases of borderline dysplasia, the co-existence of cam morphology should be considered.

4. Computer navigation-assisted arthroscopic osteochondroplasty

The planning data are transferred directly to a CT-based navigation system (Orthomap 3D; Stryker, Kalamazoo, MI). The technical details of computer navigation-assisted arthroscopic surgery have been published previously [7]. The most important and challenging aspect is point-to-point matching under fluoroscopic guidance (**Figure 5**). After matching five or six landmark points, surface matching of 40–50 points is performed. It is important to add several distal femur points to ensure accurate registration, and to add points from as large an area as possible. The final mean deviation error after registration must be <1 mm. After registration, an instrument tracker device is attached to the abrader burr. The tracker device must be fixed securely to the abrader burr, as any loosening of the device will result in variance in the navigation. Computer navigation-assisted osteochondroplasty is then initiated, during which time fluoroscopic guidance is not required.

The most notable advantage of navigation assistance is that it provides information on the actual depth and range of the resected area in real-time, seen as the tip of abrader burr (**Figure 6**). In addition, the planned resection area can also be seen as a red zone. It is, therefore, possible to accurately resect a cam lesion, without deficiency or excess. Using a pointer device, the resected region can be reliably

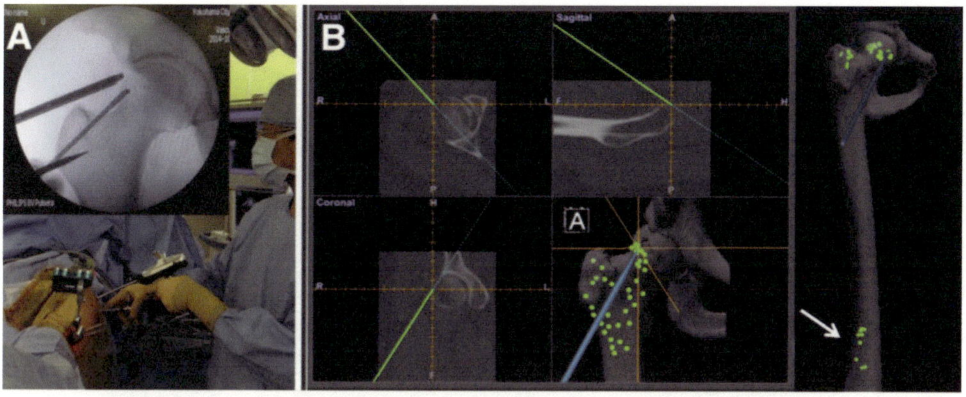

Kobayashi et al. Arthroscopy Techniques, Vol 7, No 4 (April), 2018: pp e397-e403

Figure 5.
Point matching under fluoroscopic guidance (A) and surface matching (B) during navigation system registration. Point matching is performed under fluoroscopic guidance for 5–6 landmark points (A). Thereafter, surface matching is performed without fluoroscopic guidance for 40–50 points, including on the distal femur (arrow) (B).

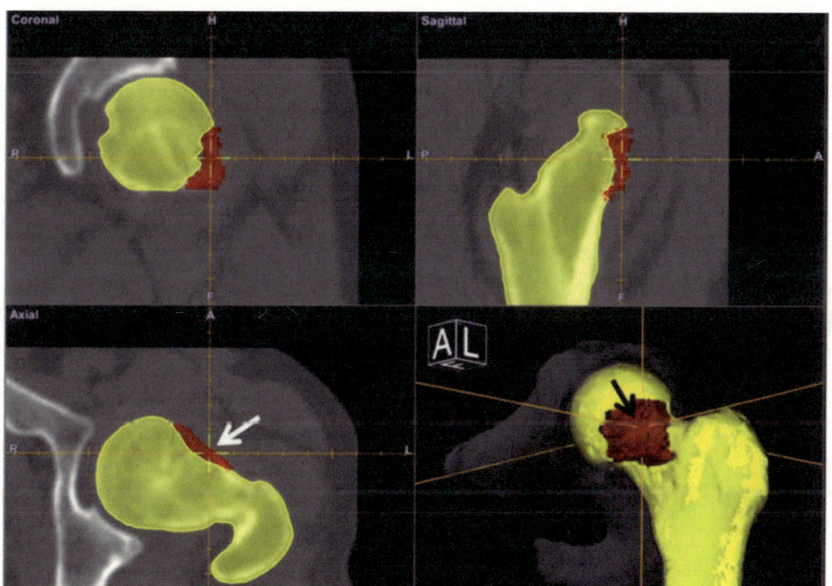

Kobayashi et al. Arthroscopy Techniques, Vol 7, No 4 (April), 2018: pp e397-e403

Figure 6.
Navigation assistance during osteochondroplasty. The center of the cross (arrow) indicates the tip of the abrader burr located in the planned resection area (red area).

verified (**Figure 7**). Occasionally, it may be necessary to use pincer resection. In these cases, it is also possible to plan the pincer resection and to use navigation assistance once pelvic registration has been completed (**Figure 8**). Particularly in pincer resection, it is difficult to identify the acetabular rim three-dimensionally by fluoroscopy, while navigation assistance can clearly identify the actual point on acetabula rim. Thus, the navigation assistance may contribute to the reduction of operative time during lower limb traction. This is important in terms of reducing the complication such as neurological disturbance caused by perineal post.

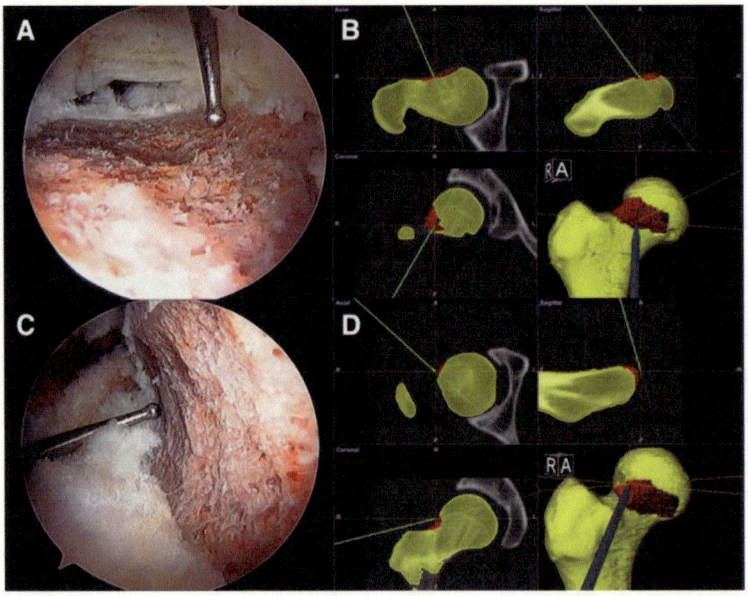

Kobayashi et al. Arthroscopy Techniques, Vol 7, No 4 (April), 2018: pp e397-e403

Figure 7.
Verification of resected area and depth using a pointer device. The pointer device indicates the distal margin of the resected area from the anterolateral portal view with the pointer via the mid-anterior portal (A), which is also identified by the computer navigation monitor (B). The lateral margin of the resected area is clearly verified from the mid-anterior portal view with the pointer via the anterolateral portal (C, D).

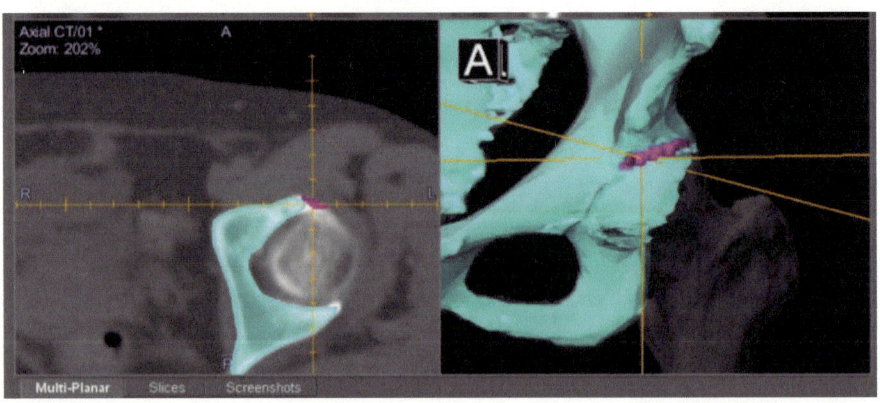

Figure 8.
Navigation assistance for pincer resection. The purple colored area shows the planned resection for a pincer lesion. The center of the cross indicates the tip of the abrader burr.

5. Postoperative evaluation

Postoperative evaluation is also possible and provides useful clinical feedback. Improvement in the maximum internal rotation angle indicates a release from the bony impingement. Ross et al. also adopted computer simulation analysis to evaluate the three-dimensional morphology of hips with residual symptoms prior to revision FAI surgery [5].

Another application of postoperative evaluation after osteochondroplasty is the assessment of mechanical bone strength by finite element analysis. This approach was used by Oba et al. to calculate changes in simulated fracture load between pre- and postoperative femur models in a clinical study of postoperative

FAI subjects [8]. The results suggested that the bone resection depth measured at the head-neck junction and transcervical reference plane correlates with fracture risk after osteochondroplasty. By contrast, bone resection at more proximal areas did not have a significant influence on the postoperative femur model strength [8]. Similarly, Alonso-Rasgado et al. concluded that resection depth should be kept to <10 mm or 1/3 of the diameter of the neck based on their finite element study [9]. These clinical implications provide valuable feedback to improve the preoperative planning of future cases (**Figure 1**).

6. Limitations and future prospects

There are several important limitations in the methodology of computer simulation. First, the bone model used in the simulation does not assess factors related to the soft tissue, including the labrum. Therefore, impingement simulation that includes consideration of the soft tissues may be required. Secondly, the simulation conditions, i.e., the variation of flexion angle, have not yet been fully established. In addition, the influence of pelvic tilt must be considered, as dynamic changes significantly influence the impingement location and simulated range of motion [10]. Currently, we use the functional pelvic plane as the reference plane; however, pelvic tilt would certainly be influenced by interventions, such as rehabilitation or surgery [11].

7. Conclusion

A summary of the preoperative assessment, planning, and navigation for arthroscopic FAI surgery using computer-assisted technology is presented. Each step of computer-assisted technology is mutually related, and it is important to comprehend this technology as a sequential flow. Although there are several limitations that need to be addressed, the notable benefits can contribute to the successful treatment of FAI.

Acknowledgements

The authors gratefully acknowledge Takayuki Oisi, Msastoshi Oba, and So Kubota for contributing related study projects.

Reprinted from [7] with permission from Elsevier.

Conflict of interest

The authors have no conflict of interest to declare.

Author details

Naomi Kobayashi[1*], Shota Higashihira[2] and Yutaka Inaba[2]

1 Department of Orthopaedic Surgery, Yokohama City University Medical Center, Yokohama, Kanagawa, Japan

2 Department of Orthopaedic Surgery, Yokohama City University, Yokohama, Kanagawa, Japan

*Address all correspondence to: naomik58@aol.com

References

[1] Bedi A, Dolan M, Magennis E, Lipman J, Buly R, Kelly BT. Computer-assisted modeling of osseous impingement and resection in femoroacetabular impingement. Arthroscopy: The Journal of Arthroscopic & Related Surgery. 2012;**28**(2):204-210

[2] Kobayashi N, Inaba Y, Kubota S, Nakamura S, Tezuka T, Yukizawa Y, et al. The distribution of impingement region in cam-type femoroacetabular impingement and borderline dysplasia of the hip with or without cam deformity: A computer simulation study. Arthroscopy: The Journal of Arthroscopic & Related Surgery [Internet]. 2017;**33**(2):329-334. DOI: 10.1016/j.arthro.2016.08.018

[3] Oishi T, Kobayashi N, Inaba Y, Choe H, Tezuka T, Kubota S, et al. The relationship between the location of uptake on positron emission tomography/computed tomography and the impingement point by computer simulation in femoroacetabular impingement syndrome with cam morphology. Arthroscopy: The Journal of Arthroscopic & Related Surgery. 2018;**34**(4):1253-1261

[4] Maquer G, Bürki A, Nuss K, Zysset PK, Tannast M. Head-neck osteoplasty has minor effect on the strength of an ovine cam-FAI model: In vitro and finite element analyses. Clinical Orthopaedics and Related Research. 2016;**474**(12):2633-2640

[5] Ross JR, Larson CM, Adeoyo O, Kelly BT, Bedi A. Residual deformity is the most common reason for revision hip arthroscopy: A three-dimensional CT study. Clinical Orthopaedics and Related Research. 2015;**473**(4):1388-1395

[6] Kubota S, Inaba Y, Kobayashi N, Choe H, Tezuka T, Saito T. Comparison of improved range of motion between cam-type femoroacetabular impingement and borderline developmental dysplasia of the hip-evaluation by virtual osteochondroplasty using computer simulation. BMC Musculoskeletal Disorders. 2017;**18**(1):3-9

[7] Kobayashi N, Inaba Y, Kubota S, Higashihira S, Choe H, Ike H, et al. Computer-assisted hip arthroscopic surgery for femoroacetabular impingement. Arthroscopy Techniques [Internet]. 2018;**7**(4):e397-e403. DOI: 10.1016/j.eats.2017.10.013

[8] Oba M, Kobayashi N, Inaba Y, Choe H, Ike H, Kubota S, et al. Mechanical strength of the proximal femur after arthroscopic osteochondroplasty for femoroacetabular impingement: Finite element analysis and 3-dimensional image analysis. Arthroscopy: The Journal of Arthroscopic & Related Surgery [Internet]. 2018;**34**(8):2377-2386. DOI: 10.1016/j.arthro.2018.03.036

[9] Alonso-Rasgado T, Jimenez-Cruz D, Bailey CG, Mandal P, Board T. Changes in the stress in the femoral head neck junction after osteochondroplasty for hip impingement: A finite element study. Journal of Orthopaedic Research. 2012;**30**(12):1999-2006

[10] Ross JR, Nepple JJ, Philippon MJ, Kelly BT, Larson CM, Bedi A. Effect of changes in pelvic tilt on range of motion to impingement and radiographic parameters of acetabular morphologic characteristics. The American Journal of Sports Medicine. 2014;**42**(10):2402-2409

[11] Oh J-S, Cynn H-S, Won J-H, Kwon O-Y, Yi C-H. Effects of performing an abdominal drawing-in maneuver during prone hip extension exercises on hip and back extensor muscle activity and amount of anterior pelvic tilt. The Journal of Orthopaedic and Sports Physical Therapy. 2007;**37**(6):320-324

Section 2

Ankle

Chapter 5

Patient-Report Outcome Measures for Ankle-Related Functionality

Tarcísio Santos Moreira

Abstract

A patient's subjective perception about his/her own functional status and also about health-related quality of life represents a challenge both for clinicians and researches, particularly in the field of rehabilitation. Clinicians often overlook the functional limitations and disability experienced by patients. Because functional limitations and disability are most important to the patient, it is essential that clinicians quantify dysfunction at this level. Client-based assessment instruments, like questionnaires, are tools suitable for comprising the domains of activity and social participation and are often the selected instrument for the assessment of health-related quality of life. In this chapter, the main aspects of such outcome measures are discussed in order to help clinicians and researchers in the selection of appropriate assessment tools in their daily practice.

Keywords: self-report measures, psychometric analysis, ankle/foot disorders, item response theory, Rasch model

1. Introduction

The main purpose of this chapter is to present a clinical and scientific perspective of the applicability of self-report outcome measures on the assessment of rehabilitation intervention designed to treat ankle/foot disorders. Some aspects about the development of these clinical tools will be briefly discussed in order to offer clinicians and scientists some criteria to better select an appropriate measure for a given clinical goal. In addition, a presentation is given of how the item response theory (IRT), by using Rasch analysis, can be used to assess such clinical measurement tools and to enrich rehabilitation data concerning clinical intervention effectiveness.

2. Patient-based outcome measures: the importance of quantifying patient's perspectives about health treatments

Throughout the history of orthopedic field, the main focus of clinical relevant outcome measures used to be those related to body structure and function, quantifying movement restrictions, such as range of motion or functional impairments like muscle strength. By this point of view, treatment goals and definitions of successful interventions captured mainly what is direct important for the healthcare professional rather than for the patient. However, what is crucial and naturally understandable for patients is functionality and disability, which brings a clear necessity

IntechOpen

to measure dysfunction at this level. Furthermore, the International Classification of Functionality (ICF) proposed by the World Health Organization (WHO) suggests that health issues should be considered by taking into account individual function, activity, and social participation. The impact that injuries, illnesses, and any other harm might have upon health, especially over functionality and quality of life, must be considered in a context of clinical evaluation in the health area.

Usually, ankle dysfunctions require the involvement of a wide variety of healthcare professionals in order to achieve excellence in recovery and functionality. This is particularly true when the treatment plan includes surgery, medications, rehabilitation program, and many other interventions carried out by different professionals. Multidisciplinary healthcare thus requires instruments that work across distinct disciplines in a sense of combining them and unifying perspectives.

The health team may have priorities that can diverge from patient-specific needs or beliefs. This may happen often because both look for a health condition from different backgrounds and starting points and this communication noise may lead to inappropriate treatment plan and can decrease patient's compliance.

Focusing on the patient, who is most interested in full recovering of his/her health, quantifying subjective perception of functional status as well as health-related quality of life represents a challenge both for clinicians and researches, particularly in the field of rehabilitation. A patient-centered or also called client-based assessment tool is needed and should meet the clinical needs of both the patient and the healthcare team, in such a way that it must be practical and accepted by everyone involved in a treatment context [1–17].

Client-based assessment instruments, like questionnaires, are tools suitable to comprise the domains of activity and social participation being commonly the selected instrument for the assessment of health-related quality of life. They have the ultimate goal of transforming subjective measures into objective data that can be quantified and analyzed. Self-report questionnaires are useful both for clinical and scientific research purposes once they combine efficiency, reliability, and low cost and, at the same time, meeting the necessity to quantify patient-centered clinical outcome measures.

3. Practical scenario: clinical use of self-report assessment tools

Every clinical outcome measure may have five goals in order to be useful in a clinical-based scenario. The acronym that exemplifies this feature is known as SMART goals and can be visualized in **Figure 1**.

3.1 Target population and purpose of the measurement tool

One way to classify questionnaires and functional scales is by their assessment application (see **Figure 2**). In this case, they can be categorized as being generic or specific. Generic questionnaires measure overall health, within biopsychosocial approach, and are intended to be applicable across a wide spectrum of diseases, interventions, demographic, and cultural subgroups. The most famous and used instrument that encompasses this properties is the 36-item short-form health survey (SF-36), which measure health-related quality of life in two main domains of mental and physical health. On the other hand, disease-specific measures aim to assess the most important traits usually affected by a condition of interest and that can be used to determine clinical improvement or deterioration. The foot and ankle outcome score (FAOS) and the American Orthopedic Foot and Ankle Society ankle-hindfoot scale (AOFAS) are both examples of condition-specific measures.

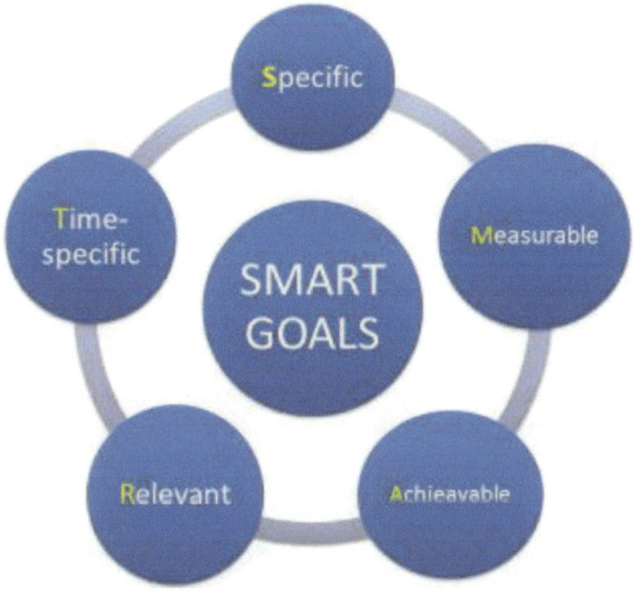

Figure 1.
SMART goals for a clinical assessment tool.

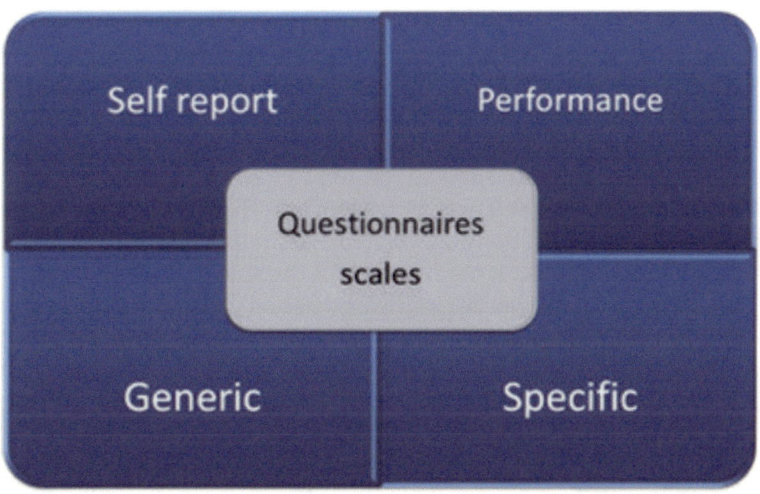

Figure 2.
Questionnaires and functional scale classification schema.

Another form in which self-report tools can be organized is in relation to the clinical function (see **Figure 2**). Within this context, they can be discriminative or evaluative instruments. The selection of one type over the other depends on the desired use of the instrument. Discriminative instruments, such as the Cumberland ankle instability tool (CAIT), can be used to identify individuals with a particular disorder, in this case, chronic ankle instability. Evaluative instruments are developed to follow up and measure an individual's change, thus assessing the effectiveness and outcome of treatment. The foot and ankle ability measure (FAAM) and lower extremity functional scale (LEFS) are examples of evaluative instruments. Information acquired from an evaluative instrument is useful only if evidence is available to support the interpretation of scores obtained in the specific population in which the instrument is intended to be used.

3.2 Practicality and feasibility

The main factors when considering practicality are the following:

1. The time expended to self-answer or to administer the questionnaire

2. The necessity of formal training or prior experience

3. Special or specific set up

4. Scoring method and use of electronic devices or software

Although patients may appear to have time to complete self-report measures in the waiting room before being seen for therapy, lengthy or numerous self-report forms may interfere with patient care. Some people may fatigue while completing self-report forms, and this fatigue could influence their responses. When selecting a self-report instrument, clinicians should pay attention on the time needed to fulfill the questionnaire. Usually, the authors report this time in scientific publications or in user's manual, when applicable. For a self-administered questionnaire, ideally no more than 10 min should be needed to answer all items.

Another important point to consider is the form of test administration. Some self-report questionnaires, especially translated versions, may require a structured interview for a proper measurement reliability. Although this procedure is likely to increase the time needed to fill in the questionnaire, it is essential to achieve an acceptable level of accuracy in measurement. Instructions for taking a test are sometimes not sufficient, and special training and experience may be necessary. Usually, there is no need for special training, but test familiarization and reading the user's guide, when applicable and suggested by the test developers, may be helpful. A great advantage of self-report measures is that no equipment or specific setups, and no professional or support staff are needed to help with the tests.

A strong point for a clinician is the importance of immediate feedback and interpretation of test result. Consequently, a scoring method that can be done manually without any software or computer assistance is desirable. It is common practice for a test's score to be attained by just summing up the individual items score and then transforming this result into a percentage. It is important to know the correct interpretation of this value, whether 100% means full function or the worst score for functionality.

Some instruments result in a single composite score or in a composite score and subscale scores for components of the item being measured. A single composite score can be desirable for communicating findings to others and for identifying people who are at risk for chronic ankle instability, for example. A composite score can be useful for discriminative instruments once a single cutoff score is an important clinical information for a diagnosis process. However, a single composite score may not represent a comprehensive analysis about physical function or ankle-related functionality for a specific task or domain. Subscale scores for components of physical function, like activities of daily living or sport related tasks, may be more useful for planning intervention and monitoring outcomes.

4. Psychometric properties

In order to ascertain that a questionnaire has proper methodological quality, information about its psychometric properties must be available. Ideally, although potentially time-consuming, information about the development of the questionnaire can sometimes be useful for a better comprehension about target population and/or medical conditions. Some author's suggest eight criteria that should be taken into account when assessing the quality of such outcome measures. These include (1) conceptual and measurement model; (2) content and construct validity; (3) reliability; (4) responsiveness; (5) floor and ceiling effects; (6) internal consistency; (7) feasibility to answer, administer, and interpret; and (8) cultural and language adaptations (translations). Reference values for each of these variables have also been suggested aiming to help clinicians and researchers in the selection and use of the clinical assessment tool that bests suits their necessity.

For the purposes of this chapter, four basic variables will be addressed in detail. They contain the minimum information needed to select and use a self-report questionnaire. They are validity, reliability, internal consistency, and responsiveness.

4.1 Validity

Content validity examines the extent to which the concepts of interest are comprehensively represented by the items in the questionnaire. It is very important to know about the following aspects regarding the development of a questionnaire for an appropriate judgment of content validity:

- **Measurement aim of the questionnaire**: it can be discriminative, evaluative, or predictive. Different items may be valid for different aims.

- **Target population**: it indicates whether the items were at the appropriate level of difficulty for the sample or the population for which the questionnaire was developed. If a questionnaire is intended to measure the functional status of patients with ankle/foot disorders, it is expected that items like *standing on tiptoes* should be much more relevant for such group than it would be for patients with knee problems. Nevertheless item's appropriateness, also the item's difficulty level, is another issue to be considered. Different populations demand different outcome measures. Ankle-related functionality of volleyball professional players, for example, requires items that measure function in a higher level of ability, with more challenging functional tasks, such as *jumping* and *landing*. In sum, a detailed description of the target population is crucial for judging the comprehensiveness and the applicability of the questionnaire for a given population.

- **Concepts:** for what the questionnaire was developed to measure. Clinicians must be aware about the relevant concepts that a questionnaire is able to measure. Quality of life, functionality, and symptoms are examples of different concepts a questionnaire may assess. These different outcome levels should clearly be distinguished and measured by separate subscales. Self-report instruments measures at the level of individual's capacity, that is, what he/she thinks they are able to do. Functional scales usually assess individual's performance, which is what he/she actually can do.

- **Item selection and item reduction:** a thorough list of potential items relating to symptoms, signs, and limitations can be gathered from literature review and input from expert clinicians (in the case of ankle-related functionality, from physicians, surgeons, and physical therapists) who treat individuals with foot and ankle-related disorders. Another important source of information is individuals with musculoskeletal pathologies within this scope. A common procedure is ask for all these people to rate each potential item from −2 (not important) to +2 (very important), and after that, reject all items with a score below +1.

- **Interpretability of the items:** completing the questionnaire should not require reading skills beyond that of a 12-year-old to avoid missing values and unreliable answers. To meet this recommendation, items should be as short as possible and, written with friendly vocabulary, understandable for a layperson out of health area. Another two points are direct questions, one attribute at a time, and direct reference about the time frame to which the questionnaire refers to.

Evidence for construct validity includes how the scores on the instrument relate to other measures of the construct, in a manner that is consistent with theoretically derived hypotheses concerning the concepts that are being measured. Construct validity should be assessed by testing predefined hypotheses. When testing expected correlations between measures, this can be called convergent validity or divergent validity when dealing with expected differences in scores between "known" groups.

Similar to construct validity is the criterion validity, which refers to the extent to which scores on a particular instrument relate to a gold standard. In a situation where there is no gold standard test or, at least, a well-established measurement tool for a given clinical condition, the analysis of criterion validity can become quite challenging. In these cases, face validity can be achieved by the process of item selection and item reduction. This indicates whether a measure appears to have been designed to measure what it is supposed to measure, in case, ankle-related functionality. Face validity, while contributing to the validity of the data obtained with a measure, is not represented by the outcome of a statistical test but by the judgment of the tester to make sure the measure has been used under similar conditions of measurement.

Evidence of validity is the first step when choosing an instrument to assess and interpret the effect of pathology and subsequent impairment on physical function, as well as to compare clinical intervention effectiveness.

4.2 Reliability

Reliability relates to score stability, and it concerns the degree to which patients can be distinguished from each other, despite measurement error. Reliability coefficients such intra-class correlation coefficient (ICC) take into account three sources of variation, that is:

- The variation among individuals, also known as interindividual variation
- The personal variation, which is the same as intraindividual variation
- At last, a variation that combines those previous mentioned, which is the error attributed to the measurement itself (measurement error)

Index like ICC is used for continuous measures and is expressed as a ration between 0 (low reliability) and 1 (high reliability). High reliability is particularly important for discriminative purposes because the difference observed in a measure should be a perfect reflection of a real change and not overlapped or shadowed by any sources of error.

Authors and test developers should provide clear information about which reliability measure they have used; if ICC is the case, the two-way random effect model is the best option for the far majority of cases. Pearson correlation coefficient is inadequate, because systematic differences are not considered. The correspondent of ICC for ordinal measures is the weighted Cohen's kappa coefficient, which is so the preferred option for such variables. In groups or samples with 50 subjects or above, the value of 0.70 is the minimum recommendation for both indexes.

4.3 Internal consistency

When adding up items with the purpose to measure, a construct is very important to know if those items are well correlated with each other and with the total score generated by them. In other words, it is highly desirable to know if the instrument is homogenous or unidimensional and so if the questionnaire as a whole measure the same concept or construct. This measure of unidimensionality is the internal consistency and is quite presumable that it should be as high or as good as possible.

There are many ways to measure internal consistency. Usually they complement each other in the process of measuring unidimensionality. The principal component analysis or the factor analysis is both very good ways to determine whether the items form only one overall dimension or not. Also confirmatory or exploratory analysis, when applicable, is useful to determine if a given group of items measure one same construct, and therefore are grouped in one scale, or if it would be better to join the items in two or more subscales. The Rasch model is also a way to measure internal consistency by using the fit statistics, which is used to assess unidimensionality, and can be simply explained as a ratio between the observed response and the response predicted by the model. This analysis is also important for evidence of construct validity, which will be better explained in the proper section ahead in this chapter.

Once the scale(s) is(are) defined, then the Cronbach's alpha is the appropriate measure of choice. Here we have two possible situations:

- A very low Cronbach's alpha indicates that there is no reason to group the items together in a same scale or questionnaire, because there are not well correlated with each other

- On the other hand, a very high Cronbach's alpha suggests that maybe there are redundant items, which means that they measure almost the same attribute of functionality. When this happens it is valuable to judge if one or more items could be removed from the questionnaire.

Cronbach's alpha should be interpreted with caution when applied to questionnaires with too many items, approximately more than 20 items. In these cases, the index is usually very high, because Cronbach's alpha is dependent upon the number of items in a scale. The reference value for adequate internal consistency when using the Cronbach's alpha range between 0.70 and 0.95.

4.4 Responsiveness

A large number of definitions and methods have been proposed for assessing responsiveness. A very good comprehensive definition for responsiveness is the ability of the instrument to detect clinically important changes in an individual's status over time even when these changes are small. This ability is the accuracy of the instrument that must be able to differentiate clinical observed changes from measurement error. Even though an instrument can capture very small changes, what really matters is to know if a change is clinically relevant. The Guyatt's responsiveness ratio (RR) does precisely this comparison by relating the variability found within the subject with between the subjects. The reference value for RR is 1.96 because this happens when the minimal important change equals the smallest detectable change.

Another adequate and common measure of responsiveness is the area under the receiver-operating characteristics (ROC) curve. It is very useful to define cutoff scores for discriminative purposes and to define injury severity. The reference value for the area under the curve is at least 0.70.

One point that impact negatively on responsiveness is the presence of floor or ceiling effects. They are considered to be present when more than 15% of respondents achieved the lowest or highest possible score. Thus, the responsiveness is limited because changes cannot be measured in these patients nor is it possible to distinguish one from another, which compromises reliability.

Limitations in measurements, such as ceiling or floor effects, can usually be avoided by selecting measures that have been demonstrated to provide meaningful information about people who are similar to those being measured. In other words, the target population of each measurement tool must be considered by matching the sample, e.g., patients with the appropriate questionnaire or functional scale.

5. "Traditional statistics" and item response theory (Rasch and factor analysis)

The Rasch model and the factor analysis constitute two ways of assessing psychometric properties of an instrument and can be, and frequently are, used in functional scales development. These two statistical procedures have the same theoretical model, which is the item response theory. The basic concept behind IRT is that the probability of choosing a response for each item is a function of both the subject's or patient's ability and the difficulty level of each item.

When applying the concepts of IRT to psychometric properties analysis, it is possible to obtain more detailed information about validity, accuracy, and targeting that helps understanding the clinical meaning of a self-report instrument. It goes beyond just looking at the final score of a questionnaire or at cutoff scores. This closer look at outcome measures like functional scales adds information to those obtained by traditional statistical tests, e.g., Cronbach alpha or ICC. IRT not only improves the methodological quality when elaborating new instruments but gives clearly insights into effects of intervention as well, whether comparing groups or the subject longitudinally.

Rasch analysis can be applied to examine instruments or assessment scales applicable in wide spectrum of disciplines, including studies in health area, education, marketing, economy, and social sciences. In the majority of evaluations, a well-defined group is selected to answer a series of predefined items. The Rasch model offers a mathematical theoretical reference by which researches that elaborate instruments are able to create comparable measures. The main point behind this model is the concept of unidimensionality, which can be summarized by the idea that useful clinical measures involve the analysis of only one human attribute at the time. In other words, it implies that the instrument measures a single latent ability. Taking a self-report questionnaire as an example, this would mean the items are organized according to their difficulty level and are placed in a single linear hierarchic scale.

The Rasch model transforms ordinal scales into interval measures. This process allows us to calibrate item difficulty and subject's ability in a same linear *continuum*, which is divided into equal intervals or *logits*. The *logits* is defined by items and works similarly as a ruler on which individuals are organized accordingly to their level of ability. The probabilistic model of Rasch analysis can be defined by the following formula:

$$Pni(x = 1) = f(Bn - Di)$$

where P is the probability of an "n" individual to succeed on a given event "i" in any trial. This probability equals to the mathematical function f of the subtraction from the "n" individual's ability "B" in relation to the "i" item's difficulty level "D." This probability can be extrapolated for multilevel items, i.e., for non-dichotomous responses. As a result of this procedure under IRT concepts, an item characteristic curve can be drawn, which represents the probability of choosing a response for each item based on the subject's or patient's ability. A typical item characteristic curve is defined by two properties: item's difficulty and item's discrimination power. Taking back the ruler analogy cited above, the difficulty of an item functions as a location index that is where in the *continuum* of ability the item works better. Hard items function with high-ability individuals as well as easy items do the same with low-ability subjects. By discrimination power, it means how well an item can separate individuals whose abilities are below or above the item location. Graphically, this property appears as the steepness of the item characteristic curve and can be interpreted as the steeper the greater the discrimination power. A flat curve means that the probability of a right answer is nearly the same with low or high levels of ability. It is worthwhile to stress out that this two properties only describe the form of item characteristic curve, and consequently how well an item function, but it cannot be used as a proof of item validity. Applying these concepts for multilevel item, Likert-like scale, for example, each answer possibility would have its own curve with distinct peaks. All the curves together should measure the spectrum of ability measured by the item.

If all items meet this probabilistic expectation, it is possible to state that the questionnaire, as a whole, assesses an unidimensional construct. This probabilistic framework constitutes the basis of Rasch model and thereby makes it possible to organize items by their difficulty level as well as by the patients' ability level, both based on the observed answering pattern.

Questionnaires should be responsive to changes in the status of the patient across the spectrum of ability. Another benefit of IRT is that it provides the amount of information that each item contributes at varying levels of ability. Easy items should provide information among low-ability levels examinees, and conversely, hard items that describe difficult tasks give information among high-ability examinees. The questionnaire final score is, therefore, the sum of all these information collected by each item, and the accuracy of it is directly proportional to the amount of information provided. The target of an evaluative instrument is to provide information across all ability ranges. Therefore, such an appropriate evaluative questionnaire should contain items that assess an individual's ability to perform activities that span from easy to more challenging ones.

The results of an item characteristic curve are valuable only when the following requirements are met:

1. Unidimensionality

    a. The questionnaire measures a single latent trait.

2. Local independence

    a. The answer for each item is independent from another item.

3. No time constraints

    a. Should be no time limit or restriction when answering the test.

4. No guessing as an answer

    a. A correct answer may not due to guessing but reflect the person's ability.

This implies that only one latent ability accounts for the individual's response for each of the items contained on the instrument, which is exactly the unidimensionality mentioned throughout this section. Both factor analysis and the Rasch model can ascertain this aspect of construct validity. Those items that did not fit to the model should be revised or eliminated accordingly with scale's goals.

6. Questionnaires and functional scales

Measures should be chosen based on whether they have been designed for and have been used with people similar to the people to be measured. For example, to assess an elite athlete's functionality after an ankle sprain, sport subscale of the foot and ankle ability measure questionnaire should provide more clinical useful information than the whole lower extremity functional scale (LEFS). This is not because one instrument is better than the other is, but because it is a better instrument selection to the target population or the right patient.

The next section shows four self-report questionnaires that are currently available for measuring ankle-related functionality. Some systematic reviews report that these instruments have very good psychometric properties and are quite useful for clinical scenarios as well as for research contexts. A brief overview for each of them is provided. For full information, we suggest to read the original studies about their development.

6.1 Lower extremity functional scale

The LEFS is a measure of activity limitation developed for musculoskeletal conditions of the lower extremity. On this scale, participants rate the difficulty in performing 20 activities of the lower extremity on a 5-point Likert scale, rating grade 0, meaning "extreme difficulty or unable to perform activity," to grade 4, meaning "no difficulty". The responses are summed to give a score ranging from 0 to 80, with 0 indicating high functional limitation and 80 indicating low functional restriction. LEFS was tested in a heterogeneous population with different lower limb conditions and was found to have high internal consistency (.96) and high test-retest reliability (r = .86) and correlated well with the physical function subscale and the physical component summary scores of the medical outcomes study 36-item short-form health survey (r = .80 and .64, respectively).

6.2 Foot and ankle ability measure

The FAAM is composed of two subscales named activities of daily living (ADL) and sports subscale, respectively. ADL subscale has 21 items and the sports subscale 8 items. Each item is scored on a 5-point Likert scale anchored by 4 (no difficulty at all) and 0 (unable to do). Item score totals, which range from 0 to 84 for the ADL subscale and from 0 to 32 for the sports subscale, are transformed to percentage scores. A higher score represents a higher level of function for each subscale.

6.3 Foot and ankle outcome score

The FAOS is a 42-item questionnaire divided into 5 subscales: "pain" (9 items), "other symptoms" (7 items), "activities of daily living" (17 items), "sport and recreation function" (5 items), and "foot- and ankle-related quality of life" (4 items). Each question can be scored on a 5-point Likert scale (from zero to four) and each of the five subscale scores is calculated as the sum of the items included. Raw scores are then transformed to a 0 to 100, worst to best score.

6.4 Cumberland ankle instability tool

The CAIT is a nine-item questionnaire designed to be a discriminative instrument of chronic ankle instability. The questionnaire is structured so that the feeling of instability is reported for different types of activities such as running, walking, hopping, and descending stairs. The nine items generate a total score from 0 to 30 for each foot, in which 0 is the worst possible score, meaning severe instability, and 30 is the best possible score, meaning normal stability. The CAIT is a reliable (ICC 0.96) instrument that can discriminate stable from unstable ankles and measure the severity of functional ankle instability.

Table 1 summarizes the main psychometric properties of each instruments reported above.

	LEFS	FAAM	FAOS	CAIT
Validity	92% of variance explained at baseline Concurrent validity r = .80 and .87, at short and medium term follow up, respectively (correlation with Olerud-Molander ankle score)	Experts and patients were involved in item generation and reduction	Item selection and reduction by patients (n = 213) Experts: not involved	CAIT and LEFS (α = .50, P < .01) and VAS (α.76, P < .01) Construct validity and internal reliability were acceptable (α = .83; point measure correlation for all items, >0.5; item reliability index, .99)
Reliability	No information	ADL subscale: ICC = .89; SEM = 2,1 points Sport subscale: ICC = .87; SEM = 4,5 points	Subscale pain, rs = .96; subscale symptoms, rs = .89; subscale ADL, rs = .85; subscale sports, rs = .92; subscale quality of life, rs = .92	ICC, 0,96
Internal consistency	α = .92 at base line; .94 short term; .90 long term.	Cronbach alpha for ADL subscale, α = .96 in stable group (n = 79); in changed group, α = .98 (n = 164) Cronbach alpha for sport subscale from a combined sample, α = .98	Subscale pain, α = .94; subscale symptoms, α = .88; subscale ADL, α = .97; subscale sports, α = .94; subscale "quality of life," α = .92	The threshold CAIT score was 27.5 (Youden index, 68.1); sensitivity was 82.9% and specificity was 74.7%.
Responsiveness	Guyatt = 1.99 AUC ROC = 0.79 (95% CI = 0.70-0.88)	MDC ADL subscale, 5.7 MDC Sport subscale, 12.3	No information	No information

Table 1.
Main psychometric properties of ankle-related self-report measures.

A. Appendix

Foot and Ankle Ability Measure (FAAM)

Please answer **every question** with one response that most closely describes to your condition within the past week.
If the activity in question is limited by something other than your foot or ankle mark not applicable (N/A).

	No difficulty	Slight difficulty	Moderate difficulty	Extreme difficulty	Unable to do	N/A
Standing	☐	☐	☐	☐	☐	☐
Walking on even ground	☐	☐	☐	☐	☐	☐
Walking on even ground without shoes	☐	☐	☐	☐	☐	☐
Walking up hills	☐	☐	☐	☐	☐	☐
Walking down hills	☐	☐	☐	☐	☐	☐
Going up stairs	☐	☐	☐	☐	☐	☐
Going down stairs	☐	☐	☐	☐	☐	☐
Walking on uneven ground	☐	☐	☐	☐	☐	☐
Stepping up and down curbs	☐	☐	☐	☐	☐	☐
Squatting	☐	☐	☐	☐	☐	☐
Coming up on your toes	☐	☐	☐	☐	☐	☐
Walking initially	☐	☐	☐	☐	☐	☐
Walking 5 minutes or less	☐	☐	☐	☐	☐	☐
Walking approximately 10 minutes	☐	☐	☐	☐	☐	☐
Walking 15 minutes or greater	☐	☐	☐	☐	☐	☐

Because of your **foot and ankle** how much difficulty do you have with:

	No difficulty at all	Slight difficulty	Moderate difficulty	Extreme difficulty	Unable to do	N/A
Home Responsibilities	□	□	□	□	□	□
Activities of daily living	□	□	□	□	□	□
Personal care	□	□	□	□	□	□
Light to moderate work (standing, walking)	□	□	□	□	□	□
Heavy work (push/pulling, climbing, carrying)	□	□	□	□	□	□
Recreational activities	□	□	□	□	□	□

How would you rate your current level of function during your usual activities of daily living from 0 to 100 with 100 being your level of function prior to your foot or ankle problem and 0 being the inability to perform any of your usual daily activities?

□□□.0 %

FAAM Sports Scale

Because of your **foot and ankle** how much difficulty do you have with:

	No difficulty at all	Slight difficulty	Moderate difficulty	Extreme difficulty	Unable to do	N/A
Running	□	□	□	□	□	□
Jumping	□	□	□	□	□	□
Landing	□	□	□	□	□	□
Starting and stopping quickly	□	□	□	□	□	□
Cutting/lateral movements	□	□	□	□	□	□
Low impact activities	□	□	□	□	□	□
Ability to perform activity with your normal technique	□	□	□	□	□	□
Ability to participate in your desired sport as long as you would like	□	□	□	□	□	□

How would you rate your current level of function during your sports related activities from 0 to 100 with 100 being your level of function prior to your foot or ankle problem and 0 being the inability to perform any of your usual daily activities?

□□□.0 %

Overall, how would you rate your current level of function?

□ Normal □ Nearly normal □ Abnormal □ Severely abnormal

Author details

Tarcísio Santos Moreira
Master of Rehabilitation Science, Universidade Federal de Minas Gerais, Belo Horizonte, Minas Gerais, Brazil

*Address all correspondence to: tarcisiosam@gmail.com

References

[1] Hale SA, Hertel J. Reliability and sensitivity of the foot and ankle disability index in subjects with chronic ankle instability. Journal of Athletic Training. 2005;**40**(1):35-40

[2] Moreira TS, Sabino GS, Resende MA. Instrumentos clínicos de avaliação funcional do tornozelo: Revisão sistemática. Fisioter Pesqui. 2010;**17**:88-93

[3] Sabino GS, Coelho CM, Sampaio RF. Utilização da Classificação Internacional de Funcionalidade, Incapacidade e Saúde na avaliação fisioterapêutica de indivíduos com problemas musculoesqueléticos nos membros inferiores e região lombar. Acta Fisiátrica. 2008;**15**(1):24-30

[4] Steiner WA, Ryser L, Huber E. Use of ICF model as a clinical problem solving tool in physical therapy and rehabilitation medicine. Physical Therapy. 2002;**82**:1098-1107

[5] Carcia CR, Martin RL, Drouin JM. Validity of the Foot and Ankle Ability Measure in athletes with chronic ankle instability. Journal of Athletic Training. 2008;**43**:179-183

[6] Vanswearingen JM, Brach JS. Making geriatric assessment work: Selecting useful measures. Physical Therapy. 2001;**81**(6):1233-1251

[7] Terwee CB, Bot SD, de Boer MR, et al. Quality criteria were proposed for measurement properties of health status questionnaires. Journal of Clinical Epidemiology. 2007;**60**:34-42

[8] Mokkink LB, Terwee CB, Knol DL, Stratford PW, Alonso J, Patrick DL, et al. The COSMIN checklist for evaluating the methodological quality of studies on measurement properties: A clarification of its content. BMC Medical Research Methodology. 2010;**10**(22)

[9] Mokkink LB, Terwee CB, Patrick DL, et al. The COSMIN study reached international consensus on taxonomy, terminology, and definitions of measurement properties for health related patient-reported outcomes. Journal of Clinical Epidemiology. 2010;**63**:737-745

[10] Martin RL, Irrgang JJ, Burdett RG, et al. Evidence of validity for the foot and ankle ability measure (FAAM). Foot & Ankle International. 2005;**26**:968-983

[11] Mokkink LB, Terwee CB, Knol DL, Stratford PW, Alonso J, Patrick DL, et al. Protocol of the COSMIN study: COnsensus-based standards for the selection of health Measurement INstruments. BMC Medical Research Methodology. 2006;**6**:2

[12] Baker FB. The item characteristic curve. In: Boston C, Rudner L, editors. The Basics of Item Response Theory. 2nd ed. College Park (MD): ERIC Clearinghouse on Assessment and Evaluation; 2001. pp. 5-11

[13] Bond TG, Fox CM. Rasch modeling applied: Rating scale design. In: Bond TG, Fox CM, editors. Applying the Rasch Model: Fundamental Measurement in the Human Sciences. 2nd ed. Mahwah (NJ): Lawrence Erlbaum Associates; 2007. pp. 219-234

[14] Binkley JM, Stratford PW, Lott SA, et al. The lower extremity functional scale: Scale development measurement properties and clinical application. Physical Therapy. 1999;**79**(4):371-383

[15] Moreira TS, Magalhães LC, Silva RD, Martin RL, Resende MA. Translation, cross-cultural adaptation and validity of the foot and ankle ability measure questionnaire. Disability and Rehabilitation. 2016;**15**:1-12

[16] Roos EM, Brandsson MD, Karlsson J. Validation of the foot and

ankle outcome score. Foot & Ankle International. 2001;**22**(10):788-794

[17] Hiller CE, Refshauge KM, Bundy AC, et al. The Cumberland ankle instability tool: A report of validity and reliability testing. Archives of Physical Medicine and Rehabilitation. 2006;**87**:1235-1241

Chapter 6

Diagnosis and Treatment of Chronic Ankle Instability

Yanyu Chen

Abstract

Ankle sprains involve up to 30% of all sport injuries. About 30% of patients may develop chronic ankle instability (CAI), which significantly limits their professional or recreational activities. The diagnosis of CAI relies on the understanding of anatomy and a thorough assessment of the patient. Imaging studies, including plain radiographs, sonography, MRI, and arthroscopic examinations, are beneficial in evaluating the extent and structures involved. Once conservative treatment has failed, surgery is indicated to restore ankle joint stability. Suture repair is sufficient, whether open or arthroscopically, if the remnant ligament quality is acceptable. Anatomical graft reconstruction is used for poor remnant quality or revision.

Keywords: ankle instability, ankle sprain, arthroscopy, Broström, reconstruction

1. Introduction

Ankle sprains are among the most common of sports injuries, and lateral ankle sprains comprise more than 80% of these [1]. Even though most of them heal well with conservative treatment, a 56–74% recurrence rate has been reported [2]. Up to 30% of patients with lateral ankle sprains end up having chronic ankle instability (CAI) [3]. The predictors of patients with single or repeated ankle sprains who may develop CAI include a grade II–III sprain [4], postural instability [5], lower limb muscle weakness or imbalance [6], and decreased ankle dorsiflexion [7].

1.1 Pathophysiology

The pathophysiology of CAI includes anatomical and/or functional deficiencies. Anatomical factors consist of pathological laxity of ankle ligaments and problematic bony structures such as hindfoot varus [8, 9]. Functional factors include neuromuscular and proprioception impairments [6, 10].

The traditional spectrum of CAI is divided to mechanical instability, which means a structurally unstable ankle and functional instability, which means a perceptionally unstable ankle. Mechanical instability of the ankle can be demonstrated manually or subjectively. Functional instability is much more difficult to evaluate; a comprehensive questionnaire is usually needed for better communication and understanding [11].

1.2 Functional anatomy

1.2.1 Bony structure

The ankle joint consists of the ankle mortise and talus. The tibial plafond forms the ankle mortise, together with the distal fibula through syndesmosis ligaments. The width of the talar dome is wider in the anterior aspect. Hence, the ankle joint is more stable in dorsiflexion position than in plantarflexion.

The stability of ankle joint will be at risk if the mortise is relatively less constrained. A posteriorly positioned fibula, either congenital or post-traumatic, may increase the anterior opening of ankle mortise and cause instability [12, 13]. The length of the fibula does not affect the stability of the ankle [14]. A decreased talar dome coverage of the tibia plafond, evaluated from plain, weight-bearing, and lateral view radiographs as well as an increased lateral radius of the talus, is linked to the development of lateral ankle instability (LAI) [13, 15].

Medial ankle instability (MAI) is less discussed in the literature. It has been reported that during arthroscopic exploration for lateral ankle instability, 20% of patients show a concomitant injury of the deltoid [16]. MAI involves the dysfunction of the deltoid ligament complex, which may cause valgus deformity of the ankle, and, vice versa, hindfoot valgus deformity carries a higher risk of developing MAI.

1.2.2 Ligamentous structure

The lateral ankle ligaments comprise of the anterior talofibular ligament (ATFL), the calcaneofibular ligament (CFL), and the posterior talofibular ligament (PTFL). The ATFL is taut when the ankle is in plantarflexion position, whereas the PTFL and CFL are taut when the ankle is in dorsiflexion position (**Figure 1**) [17].

Broström surgically opened 105 sprained ankles and reported ATFL injury in two-thirds and combined ATFL and CFL injuries in one-fourth of patients [18]. This finding suggested that the ATFL is the first-line structure against supination. The ATFL has two fascicles; the superior fascicle is positioned intra-articularly, which suggests a poor healing potential and becomes stretched in ankle plantarflexion. The inferior fascicle, on the other hand, is extra-articular and shares a common insertion with the CFL in the fibula and is not stretched in ankle plantarflexion [19].

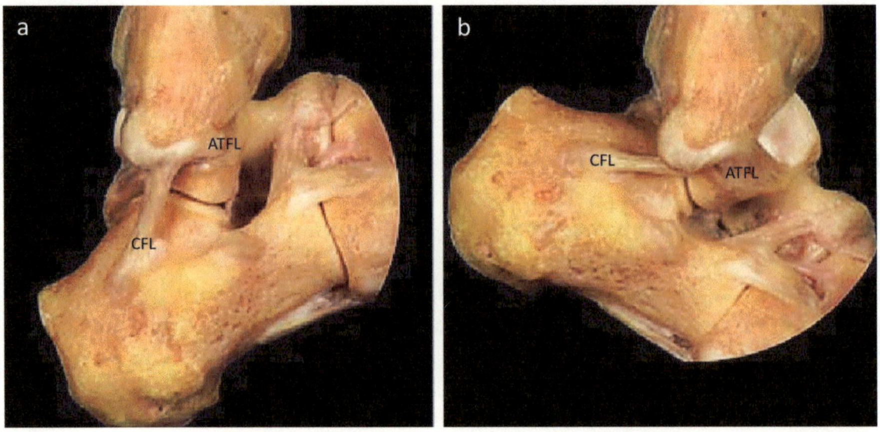

Figure 1.
Lateral view of the right ankle. The tension of the ATFL and CFL can be observed in different ankle positions: (a) dorsiflexion, (b) plantar flexion (with kind permission from Vega et al. [68]).

If the ATFL does not heal well after rupture, its laxity will result in excessive plantarflexion and supination of the ankle, which decreases the stability of the joint, increases the compensative burden of peroneal muscles, and increases the wearing of articular cartilage. Even after healing, some patients may still have lateral ankle pain and swelling despite their return of full pre-injury activity. The presence of local painful scarring, synovitis, post-traumatic weakness of peroneal muscles, and injury to the proprioception afferent fibers inside the ATFL may be the causative reasons of these residual symptoms.

The deltoid ligament is composed of a superficial layer and a deep layer. The superficial layer, which is positioned across the ankle and subtalar joint, consists of four components: the tibionavicular ligament, the tibiospring ligament, the tibiocalcaneal ligament, and the superficial posterior tibiotalar ligament [20]. The deep layer, which is thicker and positioned across the ankle joint only, consists of two components: the anterior tibiotalar ligament and the deep posterior tibiotalar ligament (**Figure 2**).

The deltoid ligament complex is composed of the deltoid ligament and the spring ligament (the calcaneonavicular ligament). The spring ligament helps not only to maintain the supination of midfoot but also to support the medial ankle structure through its connection with the deltoid ligament by the tibiospring ligament. A patient with MAI often presented with dysfunction of these two structures.

1.2.3 Neuromuscular structure

The peroneal musculature is the dynamic stabilizer of the lateral ankle joint. Lateral ankle sprains may cause injury to the ATFL as well as to the peroneal muscles. Not only can the muscular fibers be injured, the neuromuscular function can also be affected. It has been reported that the reaction time of the peroneal muscles may be delayed in patients with a history of repeated sprains, which may increase the risk of another lateral ankle sprain when the ankle lands in a supinated position [21]. This delay may be related to the deafferentation of receptors in the muscle tendon and ligaments around the ankle joint after a sprain injury [22].

Proprioception deficits are frequently encountered in patients with CAI. The dysfunction of proprioception will result in poor joint position sense, which means

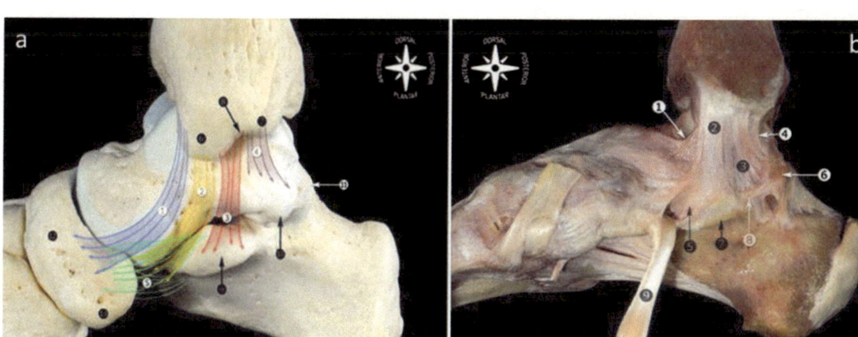

Figure 2.
Superficial and deep layers of deltoid ligament. (a) Superficial deltoid ligament. (1) Tibionavicular ligament, (2) tibiospring ligament, (3) tibiocalcaneal ligament, (4) deep posterior tibiotalar ligament, (5) spring ligament complex (plantar and superomedial calcaneonavicular ligaments), (6) anterior colliculus, (7) posterior colliculus, (8) intercollicular groove, (9) sustentaculum tali, (10) medial talar process, (11) lateral talar process, (12) navicular, (13) navicular tuberosity. (b) Deep deltoid ligament. (1) Tibionavicular ligament, (2) tibiospring ligament, (3) tibiocalcaneal ligament, (4) deep posterior tibiotalar ligament, (5) spring ligament complex (superomedial calcaneonavicular ligament), (6) medial talar process, (7) sustentaculum tali, (8) medial talocalcaneal ligament, (9) tibialis posterior tendon (from Vega et al. [68]).

in a patient with CAI that the actual ankle joint position may be much more inverted than perceived by the patient [23]. This error in joint position sense may increase the risk of lateral ankle sprains.

2. Diagnosis of chronic ankle instability

The diagnosis of CAI is mostly a clinically based diagnosis. There is no generally accepted standard of "how much laxity" is true unstable. The key idea is trying to determine whether the condition of instability could be the leading cause of the symptoms of the patient.

2.1 Presenting symptoms

The symptoms of CAI may be vague and nonspecific. Typical complaints are "insecurity" and "giving way" when running or walking on uneven ground. Patients may also complain of recurrent pain, swelling, and tenderness over medial or lateral ankle after prolonged standing or walking. Repeated ankle sprains are also a common complaint.

It should be noted that about 30% of the patients with CAI may be asymptomatic between sprains, which makes it an easily missed diagnosis [24]. Symptoms related to tendinitis, osteochondral lesion of talus, and even arthrosis of ankle joint may also be presented in patients with CAI.

2.2 Physical examinations

A comprehensive examination to check for tender points, alignment, stability, calf tension, muscle power and balance, and joint range of motion is essential for patients with potential CAI.

2.2.1 Tender points

A thorough palpation of the ankle/foot is essential in the initial evaluation of patients with CAI. An understanding of the surface anatomy is crucial for the assessment of the involved structures.

The presence of tenderness just anterior to the fibula tip indicates inflammation of the ATFL. Tenderness on the anterolateral ankle mortise that could be elicited by passive dorsiflexion of the ankle indicates possible anterolateral ankle impingement of the Bassett's ligament frequently seen in patients with CAI [25]. Bony spurs secondary to ankle arthrosis could also be a cause of anterior ankle impingement.

Tenderness on the anteromedial aspect of the ankle could indicate an osteochondral lesion of the talus or coexisting deltoid ligament injury. Tenderness on the posterolateral ankle may point to peroneal tendinitis, whereas medial foot tenderness along the posterior tibia tendon or the spring ligament is prevalent in patients with MAI.

A posteromedial ankle tenderness located anterior to the Achilles tendon indicates a possible posterior ankle impingement. A recent study showed that CAI may increase the likelihood for surgery in athletes with os trigonum syndrome [26].

2.2.2 Stress tests

Manual stress tests such as anterior drawer test and talar tilt can be positive in patients with ligament laxity, but the reliability of these tests is doubted [27].

Several modifications of the stress tests have been postulated such as the varus talar tilt test combined with an internal rotation pivot stress (VTTT with IR) and the anterior talar palpation (ATP) test [28, 29]. The VTTT with IR adds an internal rotational stress on the hindfoot with varus stress, which may better detect the rotational instability in ATFL deficiency judging from its orientation [28]. The ATP test increases the sensitivity of traditional anterior drawer test by pressing the examiner's thumb on the anterolateral ridge of the talus to better detect the anterior talar translation during the anterior draw [29].

The superficial deltoid ligament can be evaluated using the external rotation test. With the sitting patient's leg relaxed and hanging free, the degree of ankle external rotation of both legs can be compared manually. The eversion stress test can be used to assess the deep deltoid ligament by similar manner [30].

2.3 Image studies

2.3.1 Plain radiographs and dynamic radiographs

Plain weight-bearing radiographs of the ankle and foot are essential in the evaluation of patients with CAI to exclude any bony lesions and malalignment. Osseous fragments on the medial or lateral malleolar tip may indicate ligamentous or retinacular avulsion.

Dynamic radiographs can be performed manually, intraoperatively, or using a Telos stress device to demonstrate the anterior drawer test, the talar inversion, and the eversion test (**Figure 3**). For lateral ankle ligaments, a stress radiograph is considered positive when more than 5° difference compared with normal ankle or more than 10° absolute varus tilt is observed [31].

Dynamic radiographs are useful for determining the extent of instability objectively and for documentation purposes. The reported specificity of dynamic radiographs is high, but their sensitivity is low [32]. A recent study showed that preoperative stress radiographic findings do not affect the clinical outcomes of CAI after surgical treatment [33]. Therefore, the dynamic radiographs are better suited for follow-up than for diagnosis.

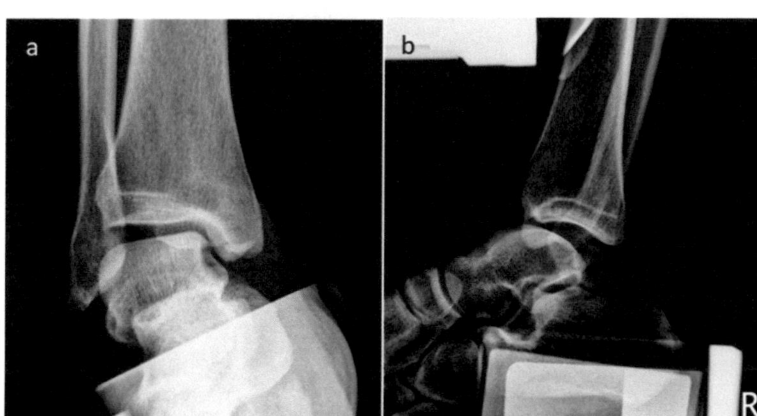

Figure 3.
Dynamic radiographs. A dynamic test using the Telos stress device showing marked varus tilt and anterior subluxation of the talus.

2.3.2 Musculoskeletal sonography

Musculoskeletal sonography allows real-time evaluation of the integrity and laxity of ligaments. It can also be used to check for tenosynovitis and periarticular synovitis of the ankle.

Evidence of an acute sprain is found when the compact fibrillar pattern of the ligament is disrupted by edema or adjacent hematoma [34]. The accuracy of sonography for an acute sprain of the ATFL and CFL is reported to be 95 and 90%, respectively [35]. Ultrasound is also highly accurate for the assessment of deltoid ligament injury after supination-external rotation fractures of the ankle [36].

In patients with CAI, the sonogram may show loss of compact fibrillar pattern and complete disorganization of the ligamentous tissue or even non-visualization (**Figure 4**) [34]. It can be used to detect small avulsion fractures in the malleolus frequently seen in patient with CAI. Stress ultrasound, either done in real-time or in combination with the drawer test, has been proposed. One study compared the relative diagnostic values of the anterior drawer test, stress radiography, stress ultrasound, and magnetic resonance imaging (MRI) using arthroscopic finding as the reference standard. The results showed 78.6% sensitivity of the anterior drawer test, 86% of the stress radiographs, and 100% of both stress ultrasound and MRI [37]. In view of the clinical availability and cost, sonography may well be the imaging tool of choice for the diagnosis of CAI [38].

The major drawback of sonography is its operator dependency and its lack of standards in the communication with other health-care professionals.

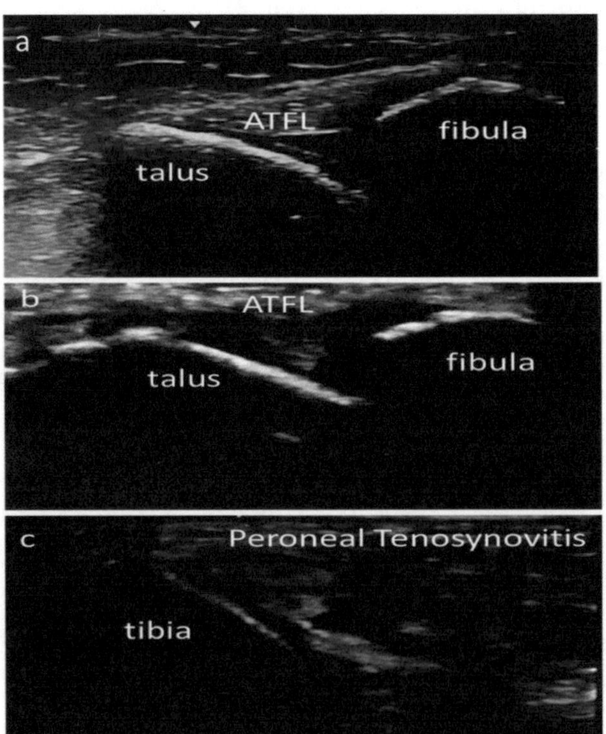

Figure 4.
Sonogram of the ATFL. (a) Normal ATFL. (b) Rupture ATFL. (c) Peroneal tendon tenosynovitis.

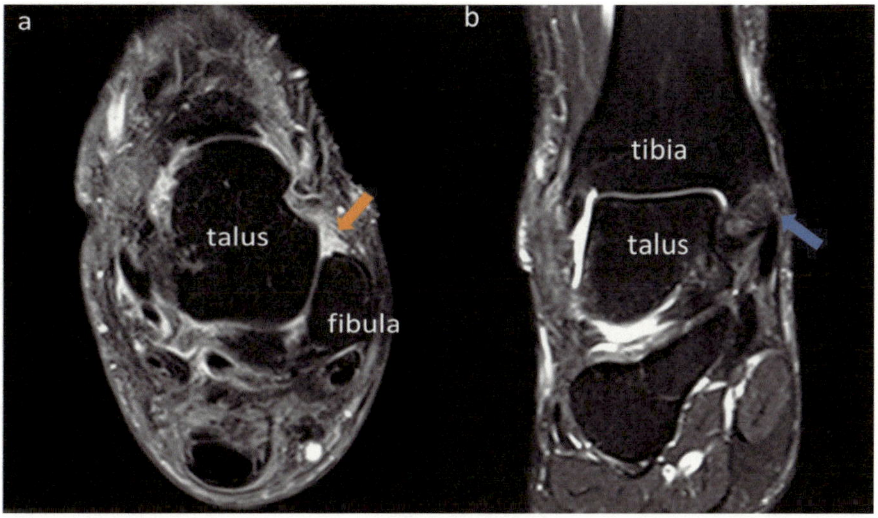

Figure 5.
MRI of injured ankle ligaments. (a) Axial view of the left ankle. The arrow points to the absent ATFL. (b) Coronal view of the right ankle. The arrow points to the injured deep deltoid ligament along with bone marrow edema in the medial malleolus.

2.3.3 MRI

MRI is useful for the evaluation of ligament integrity, thickness, and bony attachment. Normal ligaments appear as low-signal-intensity structures often surrounded by high-signal-intensity fatty tissue [39]. The ATFL is best seen in the axial plane, while the CFL and the deltoid are best seen in the coronal plane. Chronic ligament injury usually presents with morphological changes on MRI such as heterogeneous, intra-substance signals, wavy contour, thinning or elongation, and poor visualization or absence of ligament (**Figure 5**). The surrounding fatty tissue may show fibrosis with medium-signal-intensity or may show a synovitis with a high-signal-intensity [40].

The diagnostic sensitivity of MRI without contrast for ATFL rupture is reported to be 100%, whereas the specificity is only 50% [41]. MRI in combination with arthrography may improve the accuracy for diagnosing ATFL rupture to 100% [42].

MRI can also show the presence of concomitant intra- and periarticular pathologies such as osteochondral lesions, articular degeneration, bone marrow edema, tendon injury or tenosynovitis, and ankle impingement syndrome. However, MRI cannot be used to evaluate the mechanical stability of the ankle.

2.3.4 Arthroscopic examination

In the United States, nearly one-half of the patients undergo arthroscopic evaluation before ligament reconstruction [43]. Ankle arthroscopy can be performed under regional anesthesia without traction in an outpatient setting. It can provide information on the integrity, thickness, attachment, and laxity of the ligaments around the ankle joint. It can also aid in the detection of intra-articular lesions such as injuries to the articular cartilage, bony or soft tissue impingement, and syndesmosis [16, 44–47]. In ATFL and deltoid ligament injuries, the most common site of avulsion is found at the proximal insertion at the anterior aspect of fibula. The

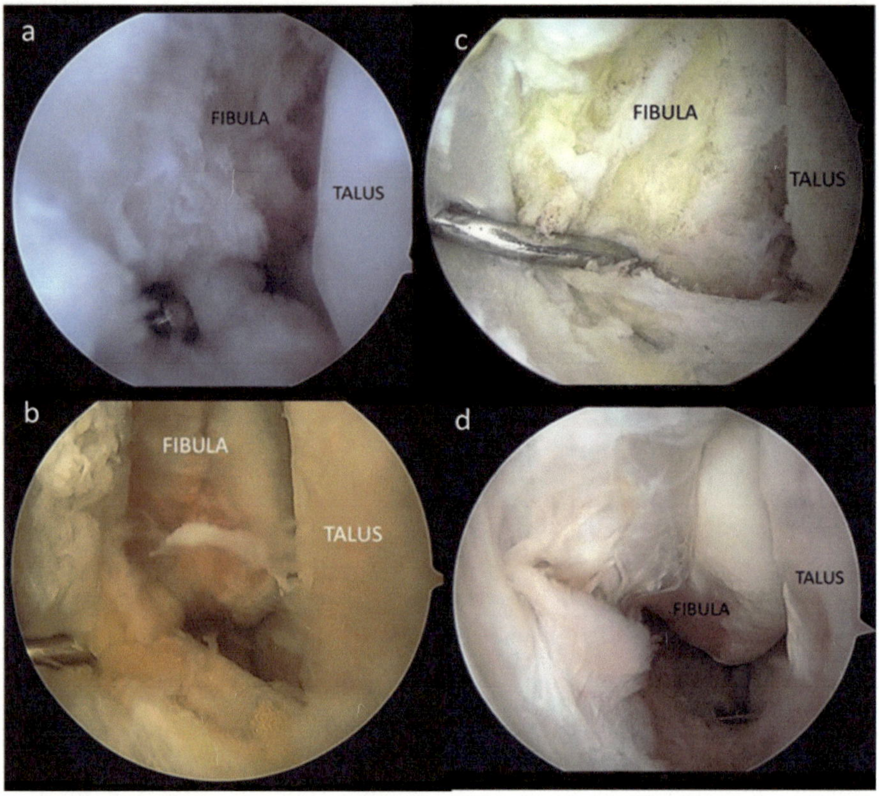

Figure 6.
Arthroscopic classification of chronic ATFL injury. (a) Grade I, distended ATFL. (b) Grade II, avulsion from fibula with decreased tension. (c) Grade III, tear and thinning with no mechanical resistance. (d) Grade IV, bald fibula (with kind permission of Thomas Bauer and the French Society of Arthroscopy [50]).

examiner can often see a bare patch of the periosteum normally covered by ligament insertion on the medial or lateral malleolus. Many authors recommended a functional arthroscopic test, which includes axial traction to quantify the tibiotalar opening, anterior drawer test, and varus and valgus tilt test [48, 49].

Using visual inspection and probe testing, injury to the ATFL can be classified in four grades (**Figure 6**) [50]:

Grade 0, which represents a normal and continuous ligament with normal thickness and tautness
Grade 1, a distended ligament with normal thickness but decreased tension by hook palpation
Grade 2, a fibular or talar avulsion (with fibrous tissue) of the ATFL, normal thickness, but decreased tension by hook palpation
Grade 3, a thin ATFL ligament with no mechanical resistance by hook palpation, with or without scar tissue
Grade 4, which shows as scar tissue with no residual ligament and leaving a bald malleolus

The author also postulated different surgical strategies according to different grading. Surgical repair and reconstruction techniques are still under debate as will be discussed later.

3. Treatment of CAI

3.1 Conservative treatment

Conservative treatment is usually reserved for the correction of proprioception deficits, balance deficits, and any static disorders. A meta-analysis showed rehabilitation attempts, including balance training, manipulation, and muscle stretch/training, which are beneficial by health-related quality of life standards in patients with CAI [51]. It has also been reported that patients with primarily functional instability are more likely to benefit from rehabilitation than patients with primarily mechanical instability [52].

3.2 Operative treatment

Operative treatment is indicated when conservative treatment failed to resolve the patients' symptoms. Patients with higher physical demands are less likely to become asymptomatic with conservative measures. Patients with mechanical instability, repeated ankle sprains, osseous fragments in the malleolar region, and limitations in on-demand activities may benefit most from operative treatment. It has been reported that patients who received surgical repair showed better muscle endurance and postural stability than patients who had conservative treatment [53].

The goals of surgery are to reestablish ankle joint stability with reduced risk of future sprains in the short term and of articular degeneration in the long term.

Several surgical techniques to reestablish ankle joint stability have been reported either by open or arthroscopic approach. These techniques can be roughly divided into two categories: suture repair and graft reconstruction.

3.2.1 Suture repair

The Broström procedure is the gold standard for patients with CAI and comes with several modifications [24]. After exposure of the remnant ligaments, the ligaments are either folded (if elongated) or reattached (if detached) back to the distal fibula using suture anchors or transosseous sutures [54]. If the quality of the remnant ligament is poor or the quality of the repaired structure is unsatisfactory, the repair can be reinforced using the nearby inferior extensor retinaculum [55]. A complication of using inferior extensor retinaculum as augmentation is that it may cause a decrease in ankle plantarflexion or pain on plantarflexion after the surgery.

Osseous fragments in the lateral malleolar region should be removed if they cause pain or are detached. However, if the fragment size is large, removal may cause a considerable soft tissue defect, which may complicate later repair [56]. Therefore, screw fixation should be considered in cases of large-sized osseous fragments.

In patients with MAI, similar procedures are used to expose, fold, and reattach the remnant ligament to the medial malleolus. If the remnant tissue quality is poor, a periosteal flap reflected from medial malleolus can be used as augmentation. The key to repair the deltoid ligament is, first, to tie the sutures with the ankle in plantigrade position and, second, to avoid sutures through the deep and superficial deltoid ligaments [27]. Sutures across both layers of deltoid ligament may cause a decrease in ankle plantarflexion or pain on plantarflexion after the surgery.

Techniques for arthroscopy-assisted or all-inside repair of both medial and lateral ankle ligaments have been proposed over many years (**Figure** 7) [57–59]. In a recent review, the postoperative functional scores, patient's satisfaction, and surgery-related complications of open and arthroscopic lateral ankle ligament repair have been compared. Excellent results were shown for both open and arthroscopic surgical procedures in the treatment of the chronic ankle instability. The higher complication rate of arthroscopic procedures relative to open ones represents a major issue; however, this does not seem to affect the patient's satisfaction [60].

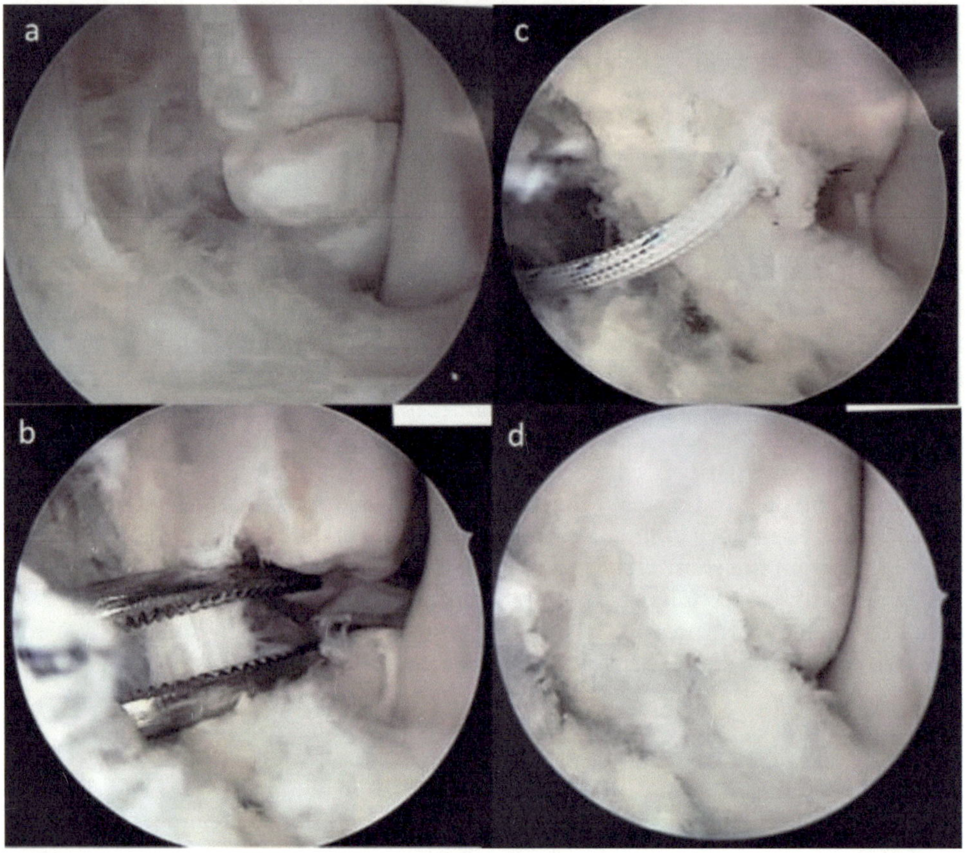

Figure 7.
Arthroscopic all-inside repair of the ATFL using suture anchor. (a) Detached ATFL and periosteum from distal fibula along with an osseous fragment. (b) Complete detachment of an osseous fragment from the fibula. (c) Application of suture anchor to fibula tip after excision of osseous fragment. (d) Reattachment of the ATFL using a suture anchor.

Weeks	Patient Mobilization	Physiotherapy
1–2	Rest, Ice, Compression and Elevation (RICE) Orthosis Walker	Lymphatic drainage
3–6	Walker Weight bearing as tolerated	ROM max PF/DF 20°/0°/10 No inversion/eversion Proprioceptive training
7–12	Orthosis if needed	Unrestricted ROM, proprioceptive training, coordination training and force

Table 1.
Postoperative treatment protocol.

3.2.2 Graft reconstruction

Using tendon grafts to reconstruct the medial or lateral ligaments is indicated when local tissue quality is poor or in case of revision surgery.

Numerous graft reconstruction techniques have been reported. They can be divided into roughly two types: anatomical and nonanatomical reconstruction.

Anatomical reconstruction is intended to reproduce the course of the ATFL and CFL as anatomically as possible. The nonanatomical reconstruction, also called peroneus tenodesis, leads to nonphysiological intra-articular pressure peaks, sacrifices a dynamic stabilizer, and causes movement restrictions. It should therefore only be used when all other treatment options have failed [61]. Recent meta-analysis concluded that nonanatomical reconstruction may abnormally increase the inversion stiffness at the subtalar level [62].

Numerous graft options have been reported including the plantaris longus tendon, hamstrings tendon, and bone-tendon-bone grafts [63–66]. These tendon grafts are fixed to the malleolus, talus, and calcaneus in various ways including the suture anchor, interference screw, and endo-button. The remnant ligaments are debrided or left in situ. There is still a lack of consensus as to which technique is biomechanically stronger or gives better functional results.

3.2.3 Postoperative treatment

Postoperative treatments of both suture repair and graft reconstruction are similar to that of acute ankle sprain. Recommendations according to the Cochrane review are listed in **Table 1** [67].

4. Conclusions

Ankle sprains are involved in up to 30% of all sport injuries with 30% of patients likely to develop CAI. These traumas can limit their professional or recreational activities significantly. The diagnosis of CAI is mainly clinically based. Sonography is cost-effective and allows real-time assessment of ligament integrity and laxity. Arthroscopic examination has the highest accuracy rate and allows direct visualization of both ligaments and intra-articular lesions.

Once conservative treatment has failed, surgery is indicated to restore ankle joint stability. Suture repair is satisfactory, whether performed open or arthroscopically if the remnant ligament quality is acceptable. Anatomical graft reconstruction is used if remnant quality is poor or a revision is required.

Conflict of interest

The authors declare no conflict of interest.

Author details

Yanyu Chen
Foot and Ankle Center, Show-Chwan Memorial Hospital, Taiwan

*Address all correspondence to: swallowfish@gmail.com

References

[1] Woods C, Hawkins R, Hulse M, Hodson A. The football association medical research programme: An audit of injuries in professional football: An analysis of ankle sprains. British Journal of Sports Medicine. 2003;**37**(3):233-238. DOI: 10.1136/bjsm.37.3.233

[2] Swenson DM, Yard EE, Fields SK, Comstock RD. Patterns of recurrent injuries among US high school athletes, 2005-2008. The American Journal of Sports Medicine. 2009;**37**:1586-1593. DOI: 10.1177/0363546509332500

[3] van Rijn RM, van Os AG, Bernsen RM, Luijsterburg PA, Koes BW, Bierma-Zeinstra SM. What is the clinical course of acute ankle sprains? A systematic literature review. The American Journal of Medicine. 2008; **121**:324-331. DOI: 10.1016/j.amjmed.2007.11.018

[4] Pourkazemi F, Hiller CE, Raymond J, Nightingale EJ, Refshauge KM. Predictors of chronic ankle instability after an index lateral ankle sprain: A systematic review. Journal of Science and Medicine in Sport. 2014;**17**:568-573. DOI: 10.1016/j.jsams.2014.01.005

[5] Munn J, Sullivan SJ, Schneiders AG. Evidence of sensorimotor deficits in functional ankle instability: A systematic review with meta-analysis. Journal of Science and Medicine in Sport. 2010;**13**(1):2-12. DOI: 10.1016/j.jsams.2009.03.004

[6] Hubbard TJ, Kramer LC, Denegar CR. Contributing factors to chronic ankle instability. Foot & Ankle International. 2007;**28**(3):343-354. DOI: 10.3113/FAI.2007.0343

[7] de Noronha M, Refshauge KM, Herbert RD, Kilbreath SL, Hertel J. British Journal of Sports Medicine. 2006;**40**(10):824-828. DOI: 10.1136/bjsm.2006.029645

[8] Crim JR, Beals TC, Nickisch F, Schannen A, Saltzman CL. Deltoid ligament abnormalities in chronic lateral ankle instability. Foot & Ankle International. 2011;**32**:873-878. DOI: 10.3113/FAI.2011.0873

[9] Morrison KE, Hudson DJ, Davis IS, Richards JG, Royer TD, Dierks TA, et al. Plantar pressure during running in subjects with chronic ankle instability. Foot & Ankle International. 2010;**31**: 994-1000. DOI: 10.3113/FAI.2010.0994

[10] Hoch MC, Staton GS, Medina McKeon JM, Mattacola CG, McKeon PO. Dorsiflexion and dynamic postural control deficits are present in those with chronic ankle instability. Journal of Science and Medicine in Sport. 2012;**15**(6):574-579. DOI: 10.1016/j.jsams.2012.02.009

[11] Gribble PA, Delahunt E, Bleakley C, Caulfield B, Docherty CL, Fourchet F, et al. Selection criteria for patients with chronic ankle instability in controlled research: A position statement of the International Ankle Consortium. JOSPT. 2013;**43**(8):585-591. DOI: 10.2519/jospt.2013.0303

[12] Scranton PE Jr, McDermott JE, Rogers JV. The relationship between chronic ankle instability and variations in mortise anatomy and impingement spurs. Foot & Ankle International. 2000;**21**(8):657-664. DOI: 10.1177/107110070002100805

[13] Bonnel F, Toullec E, Mabit C, Tourné Y. Sofcot: Chronic ankle instability: Biomechanics and pathomechanics of ligaments injury and associated lesions. Orthopaedics & Traumatology, Surgery & Research. 2010;**96**(4):424-432. DOI: 10.1016/j.otsr.2010.04.003

[14] Frigg A, Magerkurth O, Valderrabano V, Ledermann HP,

Hintermann B. The effect of osseous ankle configuration on chronic ankle instability. British Journal of Sports Medicine. 2007;**41**:420-424. DOI: 10.1136/bjsm.2006.032672

[15] Frigg A, Frigg R, Hintermann B, Barg A, Valderrabano V. The biomechanical influence of tibio-talar containment on stability of the ankle joint. Knee Surgery, Sports Traumatology, Arthroscopy. 2007; **15**(11):1355-1362. DOI: 10.1007/s00167-007-0372-2

[16] Hintermann B, Boss A, Schäfer D. Arthroscopic findings in patients with chronic ankle instability. The American Journal of Sports Medicine. 2002;**30**(3): 402-409. DOI: 10.1177/03635465020300031601

[17] Colville MR, Marder RA, Boyle JJ, Zarins B. Strain measurement in lateral ankle ligaments. The American Journal of Sports Medicine. 1990;**18**:196-200. DOI: 10.1177/036354659001800214

[18] Attarian DE, McCrackin HJ, DeVito DP, McElhaney JH, Garrett WE Jr. Biomechanical characteristics of human ankle ligaments. Foot & Ankle. 1985;**6**(2):54-58

[19] Vega J, Malagelada F, Manzanares Céspedes MC, Dalmau-Pastor M. The lateral fibulotalocalcaneal ligament complex: An ankle stabilizing isometric structure. Knee Surgery, Sports Traumatology, Arthroscopy. DOI: 10.1007/s00167-018-5188-8

[20] Milner CE, Soames RW. The medial collateral ligaments of the human ankle joint: Anatomical variations. Foot & Ankle International. 1998;**19**(5): 289-292. DOI: 10.1177/107110079801900504

[21] Hoch MC, McKeon PO. Peroneal reaction time after ankle sprain: A systematic review and meta-analysis. Medicine & Science in Sports & Exercise. 2014;**46**(3):546-556. DOI: 1249/MSS.0b013e3182a6a93b

[22] Hertel J. Sensorimotor deficits with ankle sprains and chronic ankle instability. Clinics in Sports Medicine. 2008;**27**(3):353-370. DOI: 10.1016/j.csm.2008.03.006

[23] Willems T, Witvrouw E, Verstuyft J, Vaes P, De Clercq D. Proprioception and muscle strength in subjects with a history of ankle sprains and chronic instability. Journal of Athletic Training. 2002;**37**(4): 487-493

[24] Brostrom L. Sprained ankles. VI. Surgical treatment of “chronic” ligament ruptures. Acta Chirurgica Scandinavica. 1966;**132**(5):551-565

[25] Nikolopoulos CE, Tsirikos AI, Sourmelis S, Papachristou G. The accessory anteroinferior tibiofibular ligament as a cause of talar impingement: A cadaveric study. The American Journal of Sports Medicine. 2004;**32**(2):389-395. DOI: 10.1177/0095399703258697

[26] D'Hooghe P, Alkhelaifi K, Almusa E, Tabben M, Wilson MG, Kaux JF. Chronic lateral ankle instability increases the likelihood for surgery in athletes with os trigonum syndrome. Knee Surgery, Sports Traumatology, Arthroscopy. 2018. DOI: 10.1007/s00167-018-5183-0

[27] Alshalawi S, Galhoum AE, Alrashidi Y, Wiewiorski M, Herrera M, Barg A, et al. Medial ankle instability: The deltoid dilemma. Foot and Ankle Clinics. 2018;**23**(4):639-657. DOI: 10.1016/j.fcl.2018.07.008

[28] Guerra-Pinto F, Côrte-Real N, Gomes TM, Consciência JG, Glazebrook M, Oliva XM. Varus talar tilt combined with an internal rotation pivot stress assesses the supination instability vector in lateral ankle

ligaments' injury—Cadaver study. Foot and Ankle Surgery. 2019; pii: S1268-7731. DOI: 10.1016/j.fas.2019.03.007

[29] Gomes JLE, Soares AF, Bastiani CE, de Castro JV. Anterolateral talar palpation: A complementary test for ankle instability. Foot and Ankle Surgery. 2018;**24**(6):486-489. DOI: 10.1016/j.fas.2017.05.006

[30] Hintermann B. Medial ankle instability. Foot and Ankle Clinics. 2003;**8**:723-738

[31] Chan KW, Ding BC, Mroczek KJ. Acute and chronic lateral ankle instability in the athlete. Bulletin of the NYU Hospital for Joint Diseases. 2011; **69**:17-26

[32] Cordova ML, Sefton JM, Hubbard TJ. Mechanical joint laxity associated with chronic ankle instability: A systematic review. Sports Health. 2010;**2**:452-459. DOI: 10.1177/1941738110382392

[33] Jeong BO, Kim TY, Song WJ. Effect of preoperative stress radiographic findings on radiographic and clinical outcomes of the modified Broström procedure for chronic ankle instability. The Journal of Foot and Ankle Surgery. 2016;**55**(1):125-128. DOI: 10.1053/j.jfas.2015.08.010

[34] Girish G, Finlay K, Landry D, O'Neill J, Popowich T, Jacobson J, et al. Musculoskeletal disorders of the lower limb—Ultrasound and magnetic resonance imaging correlation. Canadian Association of Radiologists Journal. 2007;**58**(3):152-166

[35] Peetrons P, Creteur V, Bacq C. Sonography of ankle ligaments. Journal of Clinical Ultrasound. 2004;**32**: 491-499. DOI: 10.1002/jcu.20068

[36] Henari S, Banks LN, Radovanovic I, Queally J, Morris S. Ultrasonography as a diagnostic tool in assessing deltoid ligament injury in supination external rotation fractures of the ankle. Orthopedics. 2011;**34**(10):e639-e643. DOI: 10.3928/01477447-20110826-11

[37] Cho JH, Lee DH, Song HK, Bang JY, Lee KT, Park YU. Value of stress ultrasound for the diagnosis of chronic ankle instability compared to manual anterior drawer test, stress radiography, magnetic resonance imaging, and arthroscopy. Knee Surgery, Sports Traumatology, Arthroscopy. 2016; **24**(4):1022-1028. DOI: 10.1007/s00167-015-3828-9

[38] Lee SH, Yun SJ. The feasibility of point-of-care ankle ultrasound examination in patients with recurrent ankle sprain and chronic ankle instability: Comparison with magnetic resonance imaging. Injury. 2017;**48**(10): 2323-2328. DOI: 10.1016/j.injury.2017.07.015

[39] Muhle C, Frank LR, Rand T, Yeh L, Wong EC, Skaf A, et al. Collateral ligaments of the ankle: High-resolution MR imaging with a local gradient coil and anatomic correlation in cadavers. Radiographics. 1999;**19**(3):673-683. DOI: 10.1148/radiographics.19.3.g99ma06673

[40] Salat P, Le V, Veljkovic A, Cresswell ME. Imaging in foot and ankle instability. Foot and Ankle Clinics. 2018; **23**(4):499-522.e28. DOI: 10.1016/j.fcl.2018.07.011

[41] Verhaven EF, Shahabpour M, Handelberg FW, Vaes PH, Opdecam PJ. The accuracy of three-dimensional magnetic resonance imaging in the diagnosis of ruptures of the lateral ligaments of the ankle. The American Journal of Sports Medicine. 1991;**19**(6): 583-587. DOI: 10.1177/036354659101900605

[42] Chandnani VP, Harper MT, Ficke JR, Gagliardi JA, Rolling L,

Christensen KP, et al. Chronic ankle instability: Evaluation with MR arthrography, MR imaging, and stress radiography. Radiology. 1994;**192**(1): 189-194. DOI: 10.1148/ radiology.192.1.8208935

[43] Werner BC, Burrus MT, Park JS, Perumal V, Gwathmey FW. Trends in ankle arthroscopy and its use in the management of pathologic conditions of the lateral ankle in the United States: A National Database Study. Arthroscopy. 2015;**31**(7):1330-1337. DOI: 10.1016/j. arthro.2015.01.020

[44] Takao M, Ochi M, Oae K, Naito K, Uchio Y. Diagnosis of a tear of the tibiofibular syndesmosis. The role of arthroscopy of the ankle. Journal of Bone and Joint Surgery. British Volume (London). 2003;**85**(3):324-329

[45] Komenda GA, Ferkel RD. Arthroscopic findings associated with the unstable ankle. Foot & Ankle International. 1999;**20**:708-713. DOI: 10.1177/107110079902001106

[46] DIGiovanni BF, Fraga CJ, Cohen BE, Shereff MJ. Associated injuries found in chronic lateral ankle instability. Foot & Ankle International. 2000;**21**(10):809-815. DOI: 10.1177/ 107110070002101003

[47] Choi WJ, Lee JW, Han SH, Kim BS, Lee SK. Chronic lateral ankle instability: The effect of intra-articular lesions on clinical outcome. The American Journal of Sports Medicine. 2008;**36**(11): 2167-2172. DOI: 10.1177/ 0363546508319050

[48] Kerr HL, Bayley E, Jackson R, Kothari P. The role of arthroscopy in the treatment of functional instability of the ankle. Foot and Ankle Surgery. 2013; **19**(4):273-275. DOI: 10.1016/j. fas.2013.06.008

[49] Guillo S, Bauer T, Lee JW, Takao M, Kong SW, Stone JW, et al. Consensus in chronic ankle instability: Aetiology, assessment, surgical indications and place for arthroscopy. Orthopaedics & Traumatology, Surgery & Research. 2013;**99**(8 Suppl):S411-S419. DOI: 10.1016/j.otsr.2013.10.009

[50] Thès A, Odagiri H, Elkaïm M, Lopes R, Andrieu M, Cordier G, et al. Arthroscopic classification of chronic anterior talo-fibular ligament lesions in chronic ankle instability. Orthopaedics & Traumatology, Surgery & Research. 2018;**104**(8S):S207-S211. DOI: 10.1016/ j.otsr.2018.09.004

[51] Powden CJ, Hoch JM, Hoch MC. Rehabilitation and improvement of health-related quality-of-life detriments in individuals with chronic ankle instability: A meta-analysis. Journal of Athletic Training. 2017;**52**(8):753-765. DOI: 10.4085/1062-6050-52.5.01

[52] Ajis A, Maffulli N. Conservative management of chronic ankle instability. Foot and Ankle Clinics. 2006;**11**:531-537. DOI: 10.1016/j. fcl.2006.07.004

[53] Lee JH, Lee SH, Jung HW, Jang WY. Modified Broström procedure in patients with chronic ankle instability is superior to conservative treatment in terms of muscle endurance and postural stability. Knee Surgery, Sports Traumatology, Arthroscopy. 2019. DOI: 10.1007/s00167-019-05582-4

[54] Cho BK, Kim YM, Kim DS, Choi ES, Shon HC, Park KJ. Comparison between suture anchor and transosseous suture for the modified-Broström procedure. Foot & Ankle International. 2012;**33**(6): 462-468. DOI: 10.3113/FAI.2012.0462

[55] Gould N, Seligson D, Gassman J. Early and late repair of lateral ligament of the ankle. Foot & Ankle. 1980;**1**: 84-89

[56] Kim BS, Choi WJ, Kim YS, Lee JW. The effect of an ossicle of the lateral

malleolus on ligament reconstruction of chronic lateral ankle instability. Foot & Ankle International. 2010;**31**(3): 191-196. DOI: 10.3113/FAI.2010.0191

[57] Nery C, Raduan F, Del Buono A, Asaumi ID, Cohen M, Maffulli N. Arthroscopic-assisted brostrom-gould for chronic ankle instability: A long-term follow-up. The American Journal of Sports Medicine. 2011;**39**:2381-2388. DOI: 10.1177/0363546511416069

[58] Vega J, Golanó P, Pellegrino A, Rabat E, Peña F. All-inside arthroscopic lateral collateral ligament repair for ankle instability with a knotless suture anchor technique. Foot & Ankle International. 2013;**34**:1701-1709. DOI: 10.1177/1071100713502322

[59] Cottom JM, Rigby RB. The "all inside" arthroscopic brostrom procedure: A prospective study of 40 consecutive patients. The Journal of Foot and Ankle Surgery. 2013;**52**: 568-574. DOI: 10.1053/j.jfas.2013.02.022

[60] Guelfi M, Zamperetti M, Pantalone A, Usuelli FG, Salini V, Oliva XM. Open and arthroscopic lateral ligament repair for treatment of chronic ankle instability: A systematic review. Foot and Ankle Surgery. 2018;**24**(1): 11-18. DOI: 10.1016/j.fas.2016.05.315

[61] Knupp M, Lang TH, Zwicky L, Lötscher P, Hintermann B. Chronic ankle instability (medial and lateral). Clinics in Sports Medicine. 2015;**34**(4): 679-688. DOI: 10.1016/j.csm.2015.06.004

[62] Cao Y, Hong Y, Xu Y, Zhu Y, Xu X. Surgical management of chronic lateral ankle instability: A meta-analysis. Journal of Orthopaedic Surgery and Research. 2018;**13**(1):159. DOI: 10.1186/s13018-018-0870-6

[63] Hintermann B, Renggli P. Anatomische Rekonstruktion der lateralen Sprunggelenkbänder mit der Plantarissehne zur Behandlung der chronischen Instabilität. Orthopade. 1999;**28**:778-784. DOI: 10.1007/PL00003667

[64] Richter J, Volz R, Immendörfer M, Schulz M. Reconstruction of the lateral ankle ligaments with hamstring tendon autograft in patients with chronic ankle instability. Operative Orthopädie und Traumatologie. 2012;**24**:50-60. DOI: 10.1007/s00064-011-0126-7

[65] Coughlin MJ, Matt V, Schenck RC. Augmented lateral ankle reconstruction using a free gracilis graft. Orthopedics. 2002;**25**:31-35

[66] Sugimoto K, Takakura Y, Kumai T, Iwai M, Tanaka Y. Reconstruction of the lateral ankle ligaments with bone-patellar tendon graft in patients with chronic ankle instability: A preliminary report. The American Journal of Sports Medicine. 2002;**30**:340-346. DOI: 10.1177/03635465020300030701

[67] de Vries JS, Krips R, Sierevelt IN, Blankevoort L, van Dijk CN. Interventions for treating chronic ankle instability. Cochrane Database of Systematic Reviews. 2011;(8): CD004124. DOI: 10.1002/14651858.CD004124

[68] Golanó P, Vega J, de Leeuw PA, Malagelada F, Manzanares MC, Götzens V, et al. Anatomy of the ankle ligaments: A pictorial essay. Knee Surgery, Sports Traumatology, Arthroscopy. 2010;**18**(5):557-569. DOI: 10.1007/s00167-010-1100-x

Chapter 7

Rehabilitation of Lateral Ankle Sprains in Sports

Rachana Dabadghav

Abstract

Lateral ankle sprains are one of the most common injuries in athletes. The rate of injury is as high as 70%. The most commonly involved ligament is the anterior talofibular ligament (ATFL), followed by the calcaneofibular (CFL) and posterior talofibular ligament (PTFL). The common mechanism of injury is inversion with excessive ankle supination in forced plantarflexion when the ankle joint is in its most unstable position. There are three grades of ankle sprains: Grade I, mild with an incomplete tear of ATFL; Grade II, moderate with a complete tear of ATFL with or without an incomplete tear of CFL; and Grade III, severe with complete tear of ATFL and CFL. Grades I and II respond well to functional treatment. Functional treatment includes RICE protocol, i.e., rest, ice, compression, and elevation. It also includes range of motion and strengthening exercises, proprioceptive training, and sports-specific exercises. Bracing and taping of the ankle joint help in preventing the sprains and also reduce the recurrence of the injury. Grade III ankle injury may be treated with surgery if the symptoms persist post functional treatment. The guidelines provided for the treatment of ankle sprains are of general validity, but each athlete is different with different needs. Hence, a personalized exercise protocol should be followed to achieve best results.

Keywords: lateral ankle sprains, athlete, sports, rehabilitation, exercise

1. Introduction

The ankle joint is the most commonly affected joint in sports of which lateral ankle sprains are the most common. The sports in which lateral ankle sprains are a frequent occurrence are football, basketball, running, volleyball, tennis, badminton, ballet/dance, etc. In many sports the rate of injury is as high as 70%. Unilateral ankle sprains are reported in 52%, whereas for bilateral ankle sprains, the number is 48%. The recurrence rate of ankle injury in athletes is 73% [1]. The incidence is high between 15 and 19 years of age with no significant difference in the gender [2].

2. Biomechanics

The lateral ankle compartment comprises the anterior talofibular ligament (ATFL), the calcaneofibular ligament (CFL), and the posterior talofibular ligament (PTFL). The most commonly injured ligament is the ATFL as it is the weakest of all three ligaments. In frequency of injury, the ATFL is followed by the calcaneofibular ligament CFL [3]. The PTFL is rarely injured as it is the strongest of all the three ligaments. The most common mechanism of injury in lateral ankle sprains is when, in forced plantar flexion, inversion occurs with excessive ankle supination. In that position the ankle joint is the most unstable. In the course of the inversion, the body's center of gravity moves over the ankle leading to ankle sprains [2]. There are three clinical grades of lateral ankle sprains [4–6].

Grade I—Mild. There is an incomplete tear of ATFL with little swelling and tenderness, minimal or no functional loss, and no mechanical joint instability.

Grade II—Moderate. Complete tear of ATFL with or without an incomplete tear of CFL with moderate pain, swelling, and tenderness over the involved structures; some joint motion is lost, and joint instability is mild to moderate.

Grade III—Severe. Complete tears of ATFL and CFL with marked swelling, hemorrhage, and tenderness. There is loss of function, and joint motion and instability are markedly abnormal.

3. Chronic ankle instability (CAI)

Athletes with chronic ankle instability give a history of two or three severe ankle sprains with the main complaint being intermittent giving out of the ankle. The athlete often complains of difficulty and apprehension on uneven surfaces. Even mild exacerbations lead to short-term dysfunction. It is characterized by residual ankle instability as a result of either mechanical ankle stability or functional ankle instability or a combination of both [6].

4. Mechanical and functional instability

Mechanical instability (MI) and functional instability (FI) are both due to recurrent lateral ankle sprains. Mechanical instability is defined as an increase in the accessory movements in the joint leading to hypermobility. Residual MI usually results from a tear or lengthening of one of the ligamentous structures supporting the joint and suggests a suboptimal healing process after injury. A lesser known phenomenon is hypomobility leading to ankle instability. Joint hypomobility can be intra-articular or extra-articular, giving rise to restricted range of motion at the ankle. Hypomobility occurs at the subtalar, talocrural joint, distal tibiofibular joint, and proximal tibiofibular joint [7, 8].

As the joint develops MI, proprioceptive changes occur, which result in alterations in defense mechanism to prevent injuries, thus leading to CAI. FI can result in balance deficits, joint position sense deficits, delayed peroneal muscle reaction time, altered common peroneal nerve function, strength deficits, a decreased range of motion (ROM), sinus tarsi syndrome, and anterolateral impingement syndrome.

5. Rehabilitation

Early mobilization of ankle sprains as compared with cast immobilization has been shown to be more comfortable as it results in less pain and provides for an earlier return to work. Cast immobilization does not improve healing compared with an active mobilization rehabilitation program and may have negative implications in relation to muscle wasting and stiffness. Functional treatment is considered better in achieving more effective mobilization and an earlier return to daily activities. Lateral ankle sprains respond well to the conservative treatment which includes initially RICE—rest, ice, compression, and elevation—followed by early mobilization. Rehabilitation focuses on restoring ROM, strength, balance, and normal gait patterns. Functional rehabilitation begins on the day of injury and continues until pain-free gait and activities are attained. Functional rehabilitation has four aspects: ROM, strengthening, proprioception, and activity-specific training. Ankle joint stability is a prerequisite to the institution of functional rehabilitation. Since Grade I and Grade II injuries are considered stable, functional rehabilitation should begin immediately.

5.1 Reduce pain and swelling

5.1.1 Rest

Rest is prescribed to avoid undue stress on the joint. It is required to reduce the metabolic demands on the injured tissue and thus avoid increased blood flow. It also helps in avoiding stress on the injured tissue that might disrupt the fragile fibrin bond, which is the first element of the repair process. Rest can be applied selectively to allow some general activity, but athletes must avoid stressful activities.

5.1.2 Ice

Cryotherapy involves a nice bath with a temperature of 4°–10°C for 12–20 min, one to three times per day, and applying an ice pack to the injured area for 15–20 min, one to three times per day. Ice therapy should be started immediately after the injury and ice application initiated within day 0 or day 1. Both have shown better results and return to full activity as compared to when the ice was applied after 48 h. Ice application should provide deep penetration to gain full benefits. Also the ice should not be held immobile in one area or frostbites may occur.

Ice application causes vasoconstriction which decreases blood flow and therefore swelling to the injured area. The lowering of tissue temperature decreases the metabolism and the chemical actions of cells and thus lowers the oxygen and nutrient needs in the affected area. Decreased blood flow limits edema; there is less histamine release and therefore less capillary breakdown than would normally be present after injury. There is better lymphatic drainage from the injured area because of the lower pressure on the extravascular fluid (**Table 1**).

Hence, the rationale of minimum 15 min of cryotherapy per treatment.

5.1.3 Compression and elevation

Compression and elevation work better in combination with cryotherapy. Compression with an adhesive bandage and a foot elevation of more than 45° is the standard prescribed treatment for lateral ankle sprains. Compression can also be

Stage	Duration (min)	Sensation
Stage 1	1–3	A cold feeling is noted
Stage 2	2–7	Burning or aching
Stage 3	5–12	Local numbness and anesthesia (decreased conductivity of regional nerve fibers)
Stage 4	12–15	Reflex deep tissue vasodilation without an increase in metabolism

Table 1.
Cryotherapy generates four stages of sensation [9].

achieved by both adhesive and nonadhesive tapes, but it is important to renew them timely as the compression wears off with time. Normally a nonadhesive tape should be renewed after 3 days, and an adhesive tape should be renewed after 5 days [10]. This prevents swelling and immobilizes the injured area which prevents further injury and thus promotes healing. Passive exercises can be started in stage 3 which is the local numbness stage in which the athlete experiences less discomfort when exercising.

5.2 Improve range of motion (ROM)

5.2.1 Range of motion exercises

Range of motion exercises include both active and passive exercises. Achilles tendon stretching should be started within 48–72 h in a pain-free range irrespective of weight-bearing status of the athlete to avoid the tissue from contracting. Self-passive stretches can also be given with the help of a towel. Next, the stretches should be extended to weight-bearing position, which can be done by standing on an inclined surface and asking the athlete to shift his/her weight forward. The stretches should be maintained 15–30 s, repeated 10 times, and should be done 3–5 times per day. Passive exercises are followed by active ROM exercises whereby the athlete can do alphabet letter exercises, i.e., drawing letters in the air both in upper and lower cases. The exercises should be done 2–3 times per hour, 4–5 times per day. Stationary biking can also be included to improve dorsiflexion and plantar flexion motion in a controlled environment while providing a cardiovascular workout for the athlete.

5.2.2 Manual therapy

Manual therapy is started within 48 h after the injury when ankle dorsiflexion is restricted. To improve range, a gentle oscillating passive joint mobilization is given. Here the talus is moved posteriorly. By the convex concave rule, when the talus is moved posteriorly, the convex talus rolls upward and slides posteriorly on the concave surface of the crux, thus improving the dorsiflexion range. In a technique described by Maitland [11], with the athlete in supine position, the affected foot is taken in the available pain-free ROM in dorsiflexion. Gentle oscillations are then given to the joint to avoid pain and spasm. The oscillations are given for 60 s, 2 or more times with a rest of 10 s taken in between.

Mobilization with movement is another technique of manual therapy suggested by Mulligan [12] which helps with increasing the ROM actively. In this technique the athlete position is high kneeling with weight-bearing on the affected limb or standing with the affected foot placed forward. In both positions the ankle is in neutral position. A padded belt is used for mobilization and is placed in such a way that the bottom of the belt is leveled with the inferior margin of the medial malleolus. The position of the mobilization belt allows the examiner to fix the talus and calcaneus with his/her hands and draws the tibia forward on the talus, thereby creating a relative posterior talar glide. Once the glide is given, the athlete actively dorsiflexes the ankle in a pain-free range. The glide should be maintained throughout the movement. Two sets of 10 repetitions, separated by a 2-min rest, are performed. Once ROM is achieved and swelling and pain are controlled, the athlete is ready to proceed to the strengthening phase of rehabilitation. Guidelines suggest that a normal ROM should be achieved within 2 weeks after injury [13].

5.3 Improve strength

Strengthening of weakened muscles is essential for a quick recovery and thus helps in preventing re-injury. An eversion to inversion strength ratio >1.0 is an important indicator of ankle sprain injury [14, 15]. Exercises should focus on strengthening the peroneal muscles because insufficient strength in this group of muscles has been associated with CAI and recurrent injury. However, all muscles of the ankle should be targeted, and all exercises should be performed bilaterally. When the training is performed bilaterally, we can expect substantial strength gains in both extremities. Strengthening begins with isometric exercises performed against an immovable object in four directions of ankle movement and is progressed to dynamic resistive exercises (isotonic exercises) using ankle weights, surgical tubing, or resistance bands.

With a structured rehabilitation program, the athlete can create continuous goals and more easily appreciate improvements. A daily adjustable progressive resistance exercise (DAPRE) strength progression, originally described by Knight [16] and later modified by Perrin and Gieck [17], can be used to create a structured progression of exercises for the athletes. The strengthening exercises should be performed with an emphasis on the eccentric component. Athletes should be instructed to pause 1 s between the concentric and eccentric phases of exercise and perform the eccentric component over a 4-s period. Concentric contraction refers to the active shortening of the muscle with resultant lengthening of the resistance band, while eccentric contraction involves the passive lengthening of the muscle by the elastic pull of the band. Resistive exercises should be performed (2–3 sets of 10–12 repetitions) in all four directions twice a day. As weight-bearing strengthening exercises, toe raises, heel walks, and toe walks should be incorporated to regain strength and coordination. Toe curling exercises with paper or towel and marble picking should also be included for strengthening of the foot musculature (**Table 2**).

5.4 Improve proprioception and balance

Once the athlete achieves full weight-bearing without pain, proprioceptive training is started for the recovery of balance and postural control. Various devices have been designed for this phase of rehabilitation. Their use in performance with a series of progressive drills has effectively returned athletes to a high functional level. As somatosensory and visual feedback is altered, the athlete must develop consistent motor patterns even with inconsistent feedback. Furthermore, the athlete can be tested under various visual and support conditions. The simplest device for proprioceptive training is the wobble board. The athlete is instructed to stand on the wobble board on one foot and shift his or her weight, causing the disc's edge to scribe a continuous circular path. These exercises can be progressed by having the athlete use different-sized hemispheres and by varying visual input. A common progression when performing balance exercise is to move from a position of non-weight-bearing to weight-bearing, bilateral stance to unilateral stance, eyes open to eyes closed, firm surface to soft surface, uneven or moving surface. Another variant is when the therapist manually moves the ankle and foot through various positions and then asks the athlete to actively and passively replicate the joint angles. This helps improving joint position sense. As the body is trained to sense directions from perturbation, sensory input is received from all parts of the body and sent to the central nervous system via afferent pathways. Therefore, conscious and unconscious appreciation is important to protect functional joint stability. Proprioception

1st set: 10 repetitions	2nd set: 10 repetitions	3rd set: 10 repetitions	4th set: 10 repetitions*
0 lbs (0 kg)	5 lbs (0.23 kg)	1 lbs (0.45 kg)	1.5 lbs (0.68 kg)
1(0.45)	1.5 (0.68)	2 (0.91)	3 (1.36)
2 (0.91)	3 (1.36)	4 (1.81)	5 (2.27)
3 (1.36)	4.5 (2.04)	6 (2.72)	8 (3.63)
4 (1.81)	6 (2.72)	8 (3.63)	10 (4.54)
5 (2.27)	7.5 (3.40)	10 (4.54)	15 (6.80)
7.5 (3.40)	11.25 (5.10)	15 (6.80)	20 (9.07)
10 (4.54)	15 (6.80)	20 (9.07)	25 (11.34)
12.5 (5.67)	18.75 (8.51)	25 (11.34)	30 (13.61)
15 (6.80)	22.5 (10.21)	30 (13.61)	35 (15.88)
17.5 (7.94)	26.25 (11.91)	35 (15.88)	40 (18.14)
20 (9.07)	30 (13.61)	40 (18.14)	45 (20.41)
22.5 (10.21)	33.75 (15.31)	45 (20.41)	50 (22.68)
25 (11.34)	37.5 (17.01)	50 (22.68)	55 (24.95)
27.5 (12.47)	41.25 (18.71)	55 (24.95)	60 (27.22)
30 (13.61)	45 (20.41)	60 (27.22)	65 (29.48)
32.5 (14.74)	48.75 (22.11)	65 (29.48)	70 (31.75)

**The athlete should proceed to the next line when he/she can lock out (complete with correct form) the 4th set 10 times.*

Table 2.
Structured strength training progression.

is useful for preventing injury in slow, moderately quick, or even quick tasks; however, it may not be adequate for forces that challenge the neuromuscular system at the highest levels. The therapist should also focus on variability of speed and intensity while training proprioception and balance (**Table 3**).

5.5 Sports-specific training

Once the distance walked by the athlete is no longer limited by pain, he/she can be put on sports-specific training or advanced training. The use of sports-specific means of training, parallel to general conditioning training, leads to considerable improvement of performance among athletes. The sports-specific training includes intricate activities like jogging which eventually progresses to running, backward running, and pattern running. Circles and figure of 8 are commonly employed patterns. These activities can also be done using ankle weight to increase the difficulty level. Star excursion balance training can also be used in which the athlete stands on the sprained ankle while using another foot to reach as far as possible in eight directions as outlined in the Star Excursion Balance Test. The exercise can consist of 8–10 rounds clockwise and counterclockwise foot reach with 3 s rest between each direction. The difficulty level can be increased by adding variations to the exercise such as with the sprained ankle (affected leg's knee) flexed, eyes opened, followed by eyes closed. At higher speed, i.e., at an angular velocity of 120°/s, the eversion to inversion ratio is >1.0, adding to the risk of injuries [19]. Hence, resistance bands can be used to strengthen the ankle musculature, i.e., training an athlete on an isokinetic machine while tying the band on the affected ankle and with the therapist holding the other end and maintaining the resistance through the movement.

No material	Ball	Balance board	Ball + balance board
Exercise 1 One-legged stance with the knee flexed. Step out on the other leg with the knee flexed, and keep balance for 5 s. Repeat 10 times for both legs **Variations** 1 2 3 4	**Exercise 3** *Make pairs. Both stand in one-legged stance with the knee flexed. Keep a distance of 5 m. Throw and/or catch a ball 5 times while maintaining balance. Repeat 10 times for both legs **Variations** 1 2	**Exercise 5** One legged stance on the balance board with the knee flexed. Maintain balance for 30 s and change stance leg. Repeat twice for both legs **Variations** 1 2 3 4	**Exercise 10** Athlete stands with both feet on the balance board. Throw and/or catch a ball 10 times with one hand while maintaining balance. Repeat twice
Exercise 2 One-legged stance with the hip and the knee flexed. Step out on the other leg with the hip and knee flexed, and keep balance for 5 s. Repeat 10 times for both legs **Variations** 1 2 3 4	**Exercise 4** *Make pairs. Stand both in one-legged stance with the hip and knee flexed. Keep a distance of 5 m. Throw and/ or catch a ball 5 times while maintaining balance. Repeat 10 times for both legs **Variations** 1 2	**Exercise 6** One-legged stance on the balance board with the hip and knee flexed. Maintain balance for 30 s and change stance leg. Repeat twice for both legs **Variations** 1 2 3 4	**Exercise 11** Athlete stands in one-legged stance with the knee flexed on the balance board. Throw and/or catch a ball 10 times with one hand while maintaining balance. Repeat twice for both legs **Variations** 1 2
Variations on basic exercises: 1. The standing leg is stretched 2. The standing leg is flexed 3. The standing is stretched and first eyes are opened, followed by eyes closed 4. The standing leg is flexed and first eyes are open followed by eyes closed 5. The standing leg is stretched and upper hand technique (throwing the ball from above the head) 6. The standing leg is flexed and upper hand technique 7. The standing leg is stretched and lower hand technique (throwing the ball while keeping the hand below the waist) 8. The standing leg is flexed and lower hand technique *This can be done by the therapist, and the athlete or the athlete can stand opposite to the wall at a distance of 5 m		**Exercise 7** Step slowly over the balance board with one foot on the balance board. Maintain the balance board in a horizontal position while stepping over. Repeat 10 times for both legs	**Exercise 12** Athlete stands in one-legged stance with the hip and knee flexed on the balance board; the other has the same position on the floor. Throw and/or catch a ball 10 times with one hand while maintaining balance. Repeat twice for both legs **Variations** 1 2
		Exercise 8 Stand with both feet on the balance board. Make 10 knee flexions while maintaining balance	**Exercise 13** Athlete stands with both feet on the balance board. Throw the ball with an upper hand technique 10 times while maintaining balance. Repeat twice for both legs **Variations** 5 6 7 8
		Exercise 9 One-legged stance on the balance board with the knee flexed. Make 10 knee flexions while maintaining balance. Repeat twice for both legs	**Exercise 14** Athlete stands in one-legged stance with the knee flexed on the balance board. Throw the ball with an upper hand technique 10 times while maintaining balance. Repeat twice for both legs **Variations** 5 6 7 8

Adapted from: The Effect of a Proprioceptive Balance Board Training Program for the Prevention of Ankle Sprains: A Prospective Controlled Trial [18].
**All the exercises done by the Athlete, can be done in pairs or the athlete can stand opposite to a wall at distance of 5 m*

Table 3.
Proprioceptive exercises (the variation and changes should be according to the athlete's requirements).

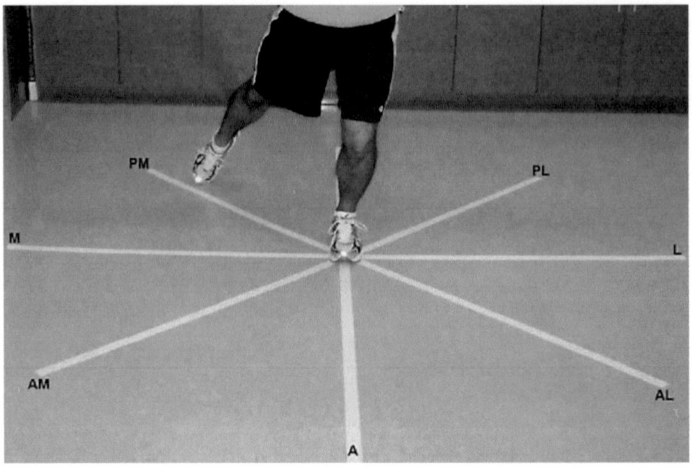

Figure 1.
Star excursion balance test [20]. Note: Star Excursion Balance Test for left-leg dominant participants (Posterior direction is behind athlete's right leg). Abbreviations: A, anterior; AM, anterior-medial; M, medial; PM, posterior-medial; P, posterior; PL, posterior-lateral; L, lateral; AL, anterior-lateral.

This should be done for 15–20 repetitions 1–2 times/day and with increasing progression. Specific training can include functional activities on various surfaces, e.g., trampoline and foam, and in water with weights. Repetitions should be 5–20, 1–2 times/day (**Figure 1**).

5.6 Criteria for return to sports

The athlete can participate fully in the sporting activity once the pain has been reduced completely. The progression should be gradual in order to stress the ligaments without causing further harm. Full participation should be allowed once the athlete has complete range of motion, 80–90% of preinjury strength and a normal gait pattern including the ability to perform sports-specific activities such as cutting and landing without any compensation due to the injury. The athlete should be able to complete a full practice without pain or swelling.

5.7 Taping and bracing

Taping and bracing the ankle can be used for prevention as well as for rehabilitation. Application of tapes and braces is helpful in the prevention of lateral ankle sprains and in the recurrence of injuries. Application of a tape or a brace increases the afferent feedback from cutaneous receptors, which lead to improved ankle joint position sense. This increased stimulation results in a more appropriate positioning of the unstable ankle and protects it from re-injury. Hence it helps improve joint position sense through proprioceptive mechanism.

a. Taping: The major role of taping is to prevent extreme range of movements and to reduce abnormal patterns of movements of the ankle. Various techniques are in use, but the most common techniques are basket weave with stirrup and heel lock and basket weave and heel lock techniques. Taping has mechanical effects: it decreases movement of inversion and plantar flexion and increases the force required for a specific displacement in inversion and plantar flexion. Taping helps in decreasing the extent of non-weight-bearing talar tilt. It also limits the full weight-bearing talar tilt. Athletes with the greatest instability benefit most from the tape. Although taping does improve mechanical instability, the restricting effect is lost after varying periods of exercise. About 40% of taping effect is lost after 10 min of vigorous exercise like jumping, pivoting, running, etc.

b. Kinesio™ taping: Unlike structurally supportive tape, such as white athletic tape, Kinesio™ tape is therapeutic in nature. It differs from the traditional athletic tape with respect to its elasticity, i.e., it can be stretched up to 140% of its original length before applying it on the skin. It provides a constant pulling (shear) force to the skin unlike traditional white athletic tape. The fabric of this tape is air permeable and water resistant and can be worn for repetitive days. The proposed mechanisms in which the Kinesio™ tape works are:

   i. It corrects muscle function by strengthening weakened muscles.

   ii. It improves circulation of blood and lymph by eliminating tissue fluid or bleeding beneath the skin by moving the muscle.

   iii. It reduces pain through neurological suppression.

   iv. It repositions subluxated joints by relieving abnormal muscle tension, helping to return the function of fascia and muscles [21].

   v. It improves proprioception through increased stimulation to cutaneous mechanoreceptors [22].

c. Bracing: Ankle bracing can make a significant contribution to preventing lateral ankle sprains. It also shows a significant reduction in the frequency of ankle sprain recurrence. Ankle braces have certain advantages over tape allowing self-application without the expertise of qualified personnel. They are convenient to apply and to remove; they are reusable, readjustable, and washable. There are nonrigid and semirigid braces. The nonrigid ones are often made of canvas or a neoprene-type material, which can easily be slipped on and off, and some are with additional lacing. The semirigid braces mostly consist of bimalleolar struts made of thermoplastic materials attached by Velcro straps. Nowadays different braces are used such as lace-up braces and the Swede-O (Swede-O-Universal, North Branch, MN) and multiple models by McDavid Sports Medical Products (Woodridge, IL); lace-up braces with straps such as the ASO (Medical Specialties, Charlotte, NC), the RocketSoc (DonJoy Orthopedics, Inc., Vista, CA), and the Ankle Brace Lock (Breg, Vista, CA); and semirigid plastic braces with strapping configurations such as the Ankle Ligament Protector (DonJoy Orthopedics, Inc.), the Universal Ankle Stirrup (DonJoy Orthopedics, Inc.), the T2 Active Ankle Support (Active Ankle, Louisville, KY) and the Ultra Ankle, and the Guardian Ankle (McDavid Sports Medical Products).

Semirigid brace like Swede-O-Universal and nonrigid brace like subtalar supports provide a better non-weight-bearing restriction in plantar flexion, dorsiflexion, and eversion than taping after 15 min of activity. A strong thermoplastic semirigid ankle brace significantly reduces talar and subtalar motions of plantarflexion, inversion, and adduction. In summary, ankle taping and bracing:

   i. Restrict ankle range of motion.

   ii. Reduce injury and recurrence rate.

iii. Improve proprioception.

iv. Lose limitation of movement after exercise.

v. Have no negative effect on most performance tests.

vi. Have little negative effect on other joints.

6. Grade III lateral ankle sprains

Grade III lateral ankle sprains occur when there is a complete rupture of both ATFL and CFL. Although the initial line of management remains a functional rehabilitation, surgery should be considered if the symptoms persist. The feeling of giving way, defined as functional instability or true mechanical instability, is frequently experienced. This can be demonstrated by provocative tests such as the anterior drawer or talar tilt (either clinically or by stress radiography). Particular attention should be directed at the diagnosis and correction of subtle subtalar instability in individuals with functional instability. Surgical repairs are aimed at the reconstruction of the normal anatomy by overlapping the existing joint capsule and lateral ligaments. The rehabilitation protocol post-surgery remains the same as that of the conservative treatment.

7. Conclusion

The early rehabilitation of lateral ankle ligament sprains focuses on gaining full recovery by starting it within 24–48 h post injury. Most of the sprains respond well to functional treatment. Rehabilitation programs should be structured and individualized. In the acute phase, the focus should be on controlling inflammation, reestablishing full range of motion and gaining strength. Once the athlete achieves a pain-free range of motion and weight-bearing, balance-training exercises should be included to regulate neuromuscular control. Advanced-phase rehabilitation exercises should focus on regaining normal function. These should include sports-specific exercises specific to the particular sport played by the athlete. While having a basic guideline to follow for the rehabilitation of lateral ankle sprains, it is important to remember that individuals respond differently to exercises. Therefore, each program needs to be modified to fit the individual's needs.

Author details

Rachana Dabadghav
Sancheti Institute College of Physiotherapy, Pune, India

*Address all correspondence to: rach.nik25@gmail.com

References

[1] Yeung M, Chan K, So C, Yuan W. An epidemiological survey on ankle sprain. British Journal of Sports Medicine. 1994;**28**(2):112-116

[2] Kobayashi T, Gamada K. Lateral ankle sprain and chronic ankle instability. Foot & Ankle Specialist. 2014;7(4):298-326

[3] Chan KW, Ding BC, Mroczek KJ. Acute and chronic lateral ankle instability in the athlete. Bulletin of the NYU Hospital for Joint Diseases. 2011;**69**(1):17-26

[4] Lynch SA. Assessment of injured ankle in the athletes. Journal of Athletic Training. 2002;**37**(4):406-412

[5] Ferran N, Maffulli N. Epidemiology of sprains of the lateral ankle ligament complex. Foot and Ankle Clinics. 2006;**11**(3):659-662

[6] Alanen V, Taimela S, Kinnunen J, Koskinen S, Karaharju E. Incidence and clinical significance of bone bruises after supination injury of the ankle. The Journal of Bone and Joint Surgery British. 1998;**80-B**(3):513-515

[7] Dananberg H, Shearstone J, Guillano M. Manipulation method for the treatment of ankle equinus. Journal of the American Podiatric Medical Association. 2000;**90**(8):385-389

[8] Hetherington B. Lateral ligament strains of the ankle, do they exist? Manual Therapy. 1996;**1**(5):274-275

[9] Hocutt J, Jaffe R, Rylander C, Beebe J. Cryotherapy in ankle sprains. The American Journal of Sports Medicine. 1982;**10**(5):316-319

[10] Capasso G, Maffulli N, Testa V. Ankle taping: Support given by different materials. British Journal of Sports Medicine. 1989;**23**(4):239-240

[11] Maitland GD. Peripheral Manipulation. 2nd ed. Sydney, New South Wales, Australia: Butterworths; 1977. p. 282

[12] Mulligan B. "NAGS", "SNAGS", "MWMS", etc. Wellington, NZ: Plane View Press; 1995

[13] Van Dijk CN. CBO-guideline for diagnosis and treatment of the acute ankle injury. National Organization for Quality Assurance in Hospitals. Nederlands Tijdschrift voor Geneeskunde. 1999;**143**(42):2097-2101

[14] Wilkerson GB, Pinerola JJ, Caturano RW. Invertor vs. evertor peak torque and power deficiencies associated with lateral ankle ligament injury. The Journal of Orthopaedic and Sports Physical Therapy. 1997;**26**:78-86

[15] Baumhauer JF, Alosa DM, Renström FH, Trevino S, Beynnon B. A prospective study of ankle injury risk factors. American Journal of Sports Medicine. 1995;**223**:564-570

[16] Knight KL. Knee rehabilitation by the daily adjustable progressive resistive exercise technique. The American Journal of Sports Medicine. 1979;7:336-337

[17] Perrin DH, Gieck JH. Principles of therapeutic exercise. In: Perrin DH, editor. The Injured Athlete. 3rd ed. Philadelphia, PA: Lippincott-Raven; 1999. pp. 123-139

[18] Verhagen E, van der Beek A, Twisk J, Bouter L, Bahr R, van Mechelen W. The effect of a proprioceptive balance board training program for the prevention of ankle sprains. The American Journal of Sports Medicine. 2004;**32**(6):1385-1393

[19] Dabadghav R. Correlation of ankle eversion to inversion strength ratio and static balance in dominant and

non-dominant limbs of basketball players. Journal of Sports Medicine and Physical Fitness. 2016;**56**(4):422-427

[20] Hardy L, Huxel K, Brucker J, Nesser T. Prophylactic ankle braces and star excursion balance measures in healthy volunteers. Journal of Athletic Training. 2008;**43**(4):347-351

[21] Kase K, Tatsuyuki H, Tomoki O. Development of Kinesio™ tape Kinesio™ taping perfect manual. Kinesio Taping Association. 1996;**6-10**:117-118

[22] Murray H. Effects of Kinesio™ Taping on Muscle Strength After ACL-Repair. Journal of Orthopaedic and Sports Physical Therapy. 2000;**30**:1-3. Available from: https://performance.nd.edu/assets/114689/kinesio_study_acl_repair.pdf [Accessed: 31 July 2019]